Traditional Chinese Medicine

Traditional Chinese Medicine

How to Maintain Your Health and Treat Illness

HENRY C. LU, PH.D.

KEY PORTER BOOKS

Library and Archives Canada Cataloguing in Publication

Lu, Henry C., 1936–
    Traditional Chinese medicine : how to maintain your
health and treat illness / Henry C. Lu.

ISBN 1-55356-017-5

1. Medicine, Chinese. I. Title.

R601.L82 2005   610'.951   C2005-901210-2

The publisher gratefully acknowledges the support of the Canada Council for the Arts and the Ontario Arts Council for its publishing program. We acknowledge the support of the Government of Ontario through the Ontario Media Development Corporation's Ontario Book Initiative.

We acknowledge the financial support of the Government of Canada through the Book Publishing Industry Development Program (BPIDP) for our publishing activities.

This book is not a substitute for medical diagnosis, and you are advised to consult your physician for specific information on personal health matters. The naming of any organization, product, resource or alternative therapy in this book does not imply endorsement by the publisher; the omission of any such name does not imply disapproval by the publisher. Neither the author nor the publisher assumes any responsibility for liability arising from any error in or omission from the book, or from the use of any information contained in it.

Key Porter Books Limited
Six Adelaide Street East, Tenth Floor
Toronto, Ontario
Canada M5C 1H6

www.keyporter.com

Text design: Jack Steiner
Electronic formatting: Jean Lightfoot Peters

Printed and bound in Canada

05 06 07 08 09 6 5 4 3 2 1

Contents

Introduction

What is traditional Chinese medicine? When and how did it originate? Based on archeological excavations, people inhabited the Chinese mainland close to a million years ago (the Pleistocene era). The fossil remains of Peking man, found in a cave at Zhoukoudian, southwest of Beijing, date back to this prehistoric era. These early people had two main objectives: first, to find food, and second, to avoid disease and cure sickness. In the struggle for survival, a need grew for some sort of medicine or health care, and out of this necessity grew the beginnings of traditional Chinese medicine in the prehistoric period.

A significant contribution to the development of traditional Chinese medicine was the evolution of the Chinese written language, starting in the so-called slave society between the twenty-first century BC and 476 BC. The transition in Chinese history from slave society to feudal society took place around the fifth century BC, and during the feudal society (476 BC to AD 618) China made significant progress in virtually all aspects of its culture, but notably in politics, economics, and philosophy. During this period of Chinese history, different types of healing arts were integrated into a coherent system of medicine with the publication of *Nei Jing*, popularly known as *The Yellow Emperor's Classic of Internal Medicine*. (I translated the *Nei Jing* into English in 1978, making it available to the Western reader in its complete version for the first time.) Any serious discussion of traditional Chinese medicine must start with this classic, for the whole history of Chinese medicine may be said to be nothing more than a series of footnotes to it.

This document has retained its importance for readers today. It contains a fascinating theory of the universe that involves health, humanity, and nature in a single, integrated system based on the two great cosmic forces, yin and yang. Yang is male, positive, active, light, heaven, and spirit, and yin is female, passive, conservative, dark, earth, and matter. All existence and activity, including health and disease, can be explained by the constant and ceaseless interaction of these two forces. In this system of dualism, these forces form a circle, one half dark and the other half light. A small light circle within the dark half is called yang within yin, and a small dark circle within the light half is called yin within yang.

Yin and yang stand in opposition to each other, but they are also two aspects of a single reality: the two forces are complementary and contrasting principles. Yin makes up for what yang is lacking, and vice versa. The wholeness of the universe, the world, and the individual human being, for that matter, would be compromised if there were a deficiency of either. Disease is a result of the two being in extreme opposition or conflict, whereas health is achieved and maintained when they are in balance. All types of therapy in traditional Chinese medicine have in common the quest for a harmonious balance of yin and yang.

All kinds of ailments can be treated by traditional Chinese medicine; some diseases may be more effectively treated by acupuncture, others are more effectively treated by herbs, and still others may be treated by food cures. In general, pain and muscular symptoms are treated by acupuncture, and skin diseases are treated by herbs. In all cases, however, it is necessary for a doctor of traditional Chinese medicine to make a diagnosis before deciding on the appropriate treatment. When a medical doctor tells a patient that there is no cure for his or her disease, it does not necessarily mean that the disease cannot be cured by traditional Chinese medicine; it only means that there is no cure by Western medicine.

A well-trained doctor of traditional Chinese medicine will select the best therapies to correct the particular illness in each patient. Acupuncture deals with a disease from the outside, while herbs and foods treat a disease from within. When the two work together, a seemingly incurable disease may be cured within a reasonable period of time.

Although many people regard acupuncture as synonymous with Chinese medicine, it is only one specialized therapy within the larger tradition. Traditional Chinese medicine includes more than a dozen forms of therapy; among them are the cures already mentioned—food cures, herbal cures, and acupuncture—but also moxibustion, Tuina (manipulative therapy), Lian Gong (exercise), Qi Gong, and Tai Chi.

Each treatment method has specific applications. If you have a common cold, for example, the treatment may be simply to eat some pungent foods—fresh ginger or green onion, perhaps—to induce perspiration; this particular treatment is a food cure. If that is not effective, you may go on to take some herbal remedies, which in most cases are successful. If you have a sprained ankle, it would be better to treat it with acupuncture, supplemented by acupressure and moxibustion. When you are recovering from knee surgery or a broken bone, Tuina therapy and various forms of exercise will bring better results. The treatment may also be combined with herbal cures or food cures to speed recovery. In the case of a chronic disease, recovery is likely to take longer so you may benefit more from Lian Gong, Qi Gong, and Tai Chi. These forms of exercise are designed to move the body in a certain way to restore inner energy and encourage recovery.

Today, Chinese doctors have combined traditional medicine with modern scientific practices. In China, there are as many hospitals of traditional Chinese medicine as there are modern hospitals of Western medicine. From the Chinese point of view, traditional medicine is on an equal footing with Western medicine. However, there are a number of basic differences between the two distinct types of medicine. For one thing, Western medicine treats symptoms, but traditional Chinese medicine treats the causes of symptoms. Second, Western medicine is more effective as first aid and surgery, whereas traditional Chinese medicine is more useful in dealing with skin and internal diseases, and chronic diseases in particular. Third, many remedies in Western medicine are based on the results of experiments on animals that may not be applicable to the human body; remedies in traditional Chinese medicine are based on successful experiences in clinical practice. Fourth, most Western chemical-based drugs are more drastic in their action and tend to produce serious side effects. Chinese herbal cures, acupuncture, and food cures are not drastic and can have long-lasting effects; they generally do not produce side effects when used properly.

Many diseases that cannot be cured by Western medicine can be successfully treated by traditional Chinese medicine. It is a fact that many patients experience instant pain relief with Chinese acupuncture. It is also a fact that traditional Chinese medicine has proven superior to Western medicine in the treatment of many diseases, particularly diseases of the skin, liver, and kidneys. Another fact is that many Western people turn to Chinese medicine to seek a solution for chronic conditions. Used in conjunction with Western medicine, traditional Chinese medicine is suitable for treating such conditions as high blood pressure, migraine, stroke, multiple sclerosis, inner ear infections, and whiplash.

From the combination of these treatments has sprung a medical philosophy and practice called holistic medicine, in which disease and its cure are related to many things, including the forms of therapy practiced in traditional Chinese medicine. Most modern Chinese hospitals have doctors of traditional Chinese medicine on the staff, and traditional Chinese medicine is even enjoying a revival among those Chinese doctors who practice modern scientific medicine. In the final analysis, the way a disease is cured is not nearly as important as the fact that the disease is cured.

When you visit a doctor of traditional Chinese medicine (TCM) for the first time, the doctor will ask you many questions about how you feel, such as whether you feel cold or hot; he or she will observe your complexion, look at your tongue, take your pulse, and ask about your symptoms and eating habits. Toward the end of the examination, the doctor may tell you the diagnosis. Before you leave the clinic, you may be given acupuncture treatment and raw herbs for decoction or herbal powder or pills. You may also be advised to take up some special forms of exercise.

The *Nei Jing* contains this statement: "A sage will prevent disease rather than cure it, maintain order rather than correct disorder, which is the ultimate principle of wisdom. To cure a disease with medicines is like digging a well when one already feels thirsty, it is like making weapons when the war has already broken out, which could be too late to do much good." The doctor of traditional Chinese medicine makes it a point to advise patients on how to maintain good health and stay free from disease.

In short, traditional Chinese medicine has the following five distinct characteristics: *simplicity*, *diversity*, *individuality*, *wholeness*, and *effectiveness*.

- The simplicity of its treatment saves time and makes self-healing not only possible but also enjoyable. For example, by following a simple recipe of food cures that you can prepare at home, you will enjoy a good meal. You can also learn how to give yourself massage when you are worn out or sick. You can also practice various forms of exercise to cure illness and promote good health.
- TCM offers a wide variety of therapies to choose from, depending on your convenience and preference. You may prefer to be treated by acupuncture rather than herbs, for example.
- TCM attaches great importance to individuality in physical makeup. Individuals are distinct from one another, both physically and psychologically, and this difference is addressed in TCM. We all have different ways of thinking, different habits, and different emotions, but in the field of health we tend to forget about the importance of individuality. To be fair, Western medicine also pays attention to individuality in its own way. For example, if you take Aspirin to relieve your headache, but it hurts your stomach, your

doctor will likely advise you to take another painkiller that does not hurt your stomach. In this way, your doctor is paying attention to your individuality. However, this is only a very tiny step toward addressing individuality. In traditional Chinese medicine, the individuality of your physical makeup is a major concern that has important bearings on the diagnosis and treatment of your symptoms. Two people suffering high blood pressure may undergo two totally different treatments, because high blood pressure in one patient may be due to a liver disorder, but in another person, it may be due to deficient energy and blood. Your headache may be caused by a common cold, but someone else's headache may be caused by a stomach imbalance, which should be treated differently.

- TCM focuses on the whole body instead of its parts. When making a diagnosis, a doctor of traditional Chinese medicine is concerned with the whole person. The doctor does not treat your stomach at the expense of your liver or vice versa, nor does the doctor treat your arthritis with drugs that cause damage to your heart. The doctor focuses on physical and psychological wholeness as key indicators of health and disease. Included in the procedure are questioning the patient, making tongue and pulse diagnoses, coupled with itemizing current symptoms and recording a detailed history. This procedure allows the doctor to piece together the patterns of imbalance, which are used to formulate a diagnosis and recommend treatment specific to the individual patient. Traditional Chinese medicine is not aimed at relieving symptoms on a piecemeal basis, but rather, it directs its attention to treating the underlying cause of the disease and thus returns the body to its balanced and harmonious state.

- The effectiveness of TCM is impressive. Recent studies in the United States, Canada, Australia, and Europe demonstrate the effectiveness and increasingly widespread use of TCM around the world. Most of the clinical studies have concentrated on acupuncture.

  According to the U.S. National Institutes of Health Conference on Acupuncture in 1997, acupuncture is widely practiced in the United States for relief or prevention of pain and various other health conditions. According to the "Consensus Development Conference Statement," 1 million Americans currently receive acupuncture treatment each year. Clinical studies demonstrate the efficacy of acupuncture in postoperative and chemotherapy nausea and vomiting and postoperative dental pain. In addition to its use as an analgesic, there is also clinical evidence that acupuncture affects a range of physiological functions, and benefits hypertension and other cardiovascular disorders, asthma and bronchospasm, digestive disorders, obstetrics, and drug addiction. The World Health Organization lists more than forty conditions for which acupuncture is effective.

CHAPTER 1

Causes of Diseases and Treatment Strategies

When yang wins a victory, there will be fever. When yin wins a victory, there will be chills. ——NEI JING

What causes disease? In Western medicine, germs and viruses are considered to be the primary culprits, but in traditional Chinese medicine disease is thought to be caused by disharmonies within the body or between the body and the environment. It is the result of a struggle between hostile forces and body energy, not unlike the struggle between germs or viruses and the immune system in Western medicine.

The causes of disease in traditional Chinese medicine are divided into three basic categories. First, there are external causes, which include six atmospheric or climatic forces: wind, cold, summer heat, dampness, dryness, and fire. The second category is internal causes, which include seven emotions: joy, anger, worry, thought, sadness, fear, and shock. Third, there are two other causes, which are neither internal nor external: fatigue and foods.

Six atmospheric forces as external causes

The six atmospheric forces are considered hostile when they cause disease in the body. When they act as positive forces, they contribute to body energy.

WIND

How does wind cause disease? Wind—air in motion—is a natural phenomenon in the atmosphere. Wind usually helps to maintain good health. When we feel hot, for example, we need wind to cool the body. We leave the windows open, particularly in the heat of summer, because we need fresh air, which will be carried in by the wind. Therefore, as a natural atmospheric energy, wind is essential to human health. But wind may be good or bad for the health, depending on the circumstances. For example, a cold wind can create a chill in the body, making you susceptible to a cold or even pneumonia. When wind causes disease, it becomes harmful to the human body, and is regarded as a hostile atmospheric force to be avoided.

COLD

When the body is under attack by cold, we experience fever, absence of perspiration, headache, and pain in the body. When cold attacks the digestive system, it will cause intestinal rumbling, diarrhea, and abdominal pain. The kidneys are most susceptible to an attack of cold; when the kidneys are under attack, other symptoms such as lower back pain and cold feet can develop.

SUMMER HEAT

When the body is under attack by summer heat, we experience high fever, thirst, and profuse perspiration. Moreover, summer heat sucks moisture and water from the body, which is why you will feel extremely thirsty and exhausted due to lack of body fluids when you are under attack by the heat. You may also have a dry mouth and lips, constipation due to dry intestines, and produce scanty urine due to a shortage of water in the body. Among the internal organs, the heart is most susceptible to the attack of summer heat; when summer heat attacks the heart, it may cause eye infections, thirst, nosebleeds, vomiting of blood, and, in severe cases, loss of consciousness.

DAMPNESS

When late summer rains make the ground very damp and at the same time the weather becomes cooler, moisture on the ground cannot evaporate as quickly as it did in early and midsummer. When you walk in the rain, sleep on damp ground, live in a damp environment, wear wet clothes or swim a lot, you become an easy target of attack by dampness. Blisters, water retention with puffiness, and diarrhea are all caused by dampness.

Many familiar conditions are associated with damp. The skin disease known as eczema, which is characterized by pus-filled lesions, is called "damp rash" in the Chinese language because it is primarily caused by dampness invading the skin. Coughing watery mucus, panting, and a congested chest are called "damp phlegm obstructing the lungs." Gurgling in the intestine is called "stoppage of dampness in the middle region." Puffiness with water retention in the whole body and difficult urination are called "flooding of dampness." The pain of rheumatism and arthritis that stays in the same spot are called "damp rheumatism" or "damp arthritis." Dampness attacks the joints, because it flows into the joints easily like water. Patients with rheumatism, arthritis, or osteoarthritis (a degenerative joint disease) caused by dampness often experience more severe symptoms when humidity is high.

DRYNESS

Dryness is the dominant energy in autumn when humidity in the atmosphere is low. When you are under attack by dryness, you may develop such symptoms as a dry cough, sore throat with dryness, dry skin, dry nose, thirst, scanty urine, and constipation with dry stools. These are all called "autumn dryness" in traditional Chinese medicine, because such symptoms most frequently occur in autumn and are due to the dryness in the atmosphere during that season.

FIRE

The human body needs fire to maintain normal body temperature. But when this force is too strong, it can cause fever. You may suffer from a common cold with low fever at the beginning. If the fever is allowed to drag on, the cold can develop into meningitis (inflammation of the membranes of the spinal cord or brain). When you are under stress for too long, you might accumulate internal heat that eventually causes insomnia, lumbago, cough, or asthma. This is called "emotions transform into fire."

Fire speeds up the rate of metabolism so that your body consumes more energy than usual, correspondingly reducing the quantity of energy left in your body. A typical example can be seen in hyperthyroidism, a hyperfunctioning of the thyroid gland in which the metabolic rate speeds up, resulting in an increased demand for food. Hyperthyroidism itself is caused by fire that consumes body fluids and eats up body energy. Although exceptions exist, most consumptive diseases are caused by fire, including hyperthyroidism, tuberculosis, fever, and many forms of cancers; such diseases consume a great deal of body fluids and body energy, weakening the body.

How does fire produce toxic effects? At the beginning, fire consumes body fluids, creating a shortage of fluids in the body. As time goes on, the shortage of body fluids may reach the stage where the body can no longer function normally, with the result that fire takes over. Symptoms caused by toxic fire are characterized by burning sensations with pain. Most cases of infection and inflammation fall within this category, including infection of the eyes, kidneys (nephritis), or throat; inflammation of the lungs (pneumonia); and infections of the urinary system. Chemotherapy and radiation therapy used to treat cancers very often produce toxic fire in the body, which is why many cancer patients complain about nausea and sore throat.

All five atmospheric forces can be transformed into fire to cause disease, but this can happen more easily when body fluids are in short supply, a condition called "yin deficiency." When the other five atmospheric forces are transformed into fire mainly because of a yin deficiency in the body, it is called "fire of deficiency"; when fire is caused primarily by the strength of the other five atmospheric forces, the condition is called "fire of excess."

Seven emotions as internal causes

Unlike animals, human beings have emotions that affect their thoughts and actions. An example of how emotion can influence physiological activities can be seen in the nursing mother: When a nursing mother is irritable during breast-feeding, milk secretion decreases or stops. Another example is the fact that the mortality rate among cancer patients who are constantly in great emotional stress is much higher than for other cancer patients.

When you are depressed, you may feel like "a candle guttering in the wind that won't last the night," as the Chinese saying goes. Various symptoms may appear, such as poor memory, loss of appetite, and low energy. Depression can also speed up the aging process. It is not uncommon for a politician to die suddenly after losing an election or for a person to die shortly after the loss of his or her beloved. All such incidents point to the connection between emotions and life expectancy. No system of medicine has put as much emphasis on emotions as does traditional Chinese medicine.

The seven basic emotions that can cause disease are *joy*, *anger*, *worry*, *thought*, *sadness*, *fear*, and *shock*. Each of these emotions has an impact on a specific organ. However, it is only when these emotions exceed a normal range or run out of control that they begin to cause disease. Excessive joy, excessive anger, excessive worry, concentrated thought, excessive sadness, persistent fear, and sudden shock will make themselves felt by causing disease.

Excessive anger is harmful to the liver, being overjoyed is harmful to the heart, concentrated thought is harmful to the spleen, too much worry and sadness are harmful to the lungs, and persistent fear and sudden shock are harmful to the kidneys. In traditional Chinese medicine, it is thought that emotions have an impact on internal organs because they disturb the energy balance in those organs. For example, when you are angry, the energy of your liver rushes upward to cause various symptoms in the head, including headache, high blood pressure, and stroke in severe cases, which is why, in extreme cases, a person may die after an angry outburst.

People sometimes say, "I was worried to death about you." Even though they do not mean it literally, they are not far wrong. When you are worried about something, you most likely begin to lose your appetite or suffer indigestion. In a study conducted in China, patients with neurasthenia (a disease marked by symptoms such as chronic fatigue and sleeplessness) were divided into two groups according to the state of their emotions. Those patients considered emotionally fit were put into the first group, and those who were emotionally unstable were put into the second group. In a given period of time, 97 percent of patients in the first group recovered from their illness while only 5 percent in the second group recovered during the same period.

When you experience any of these basic emotions to an excessive degree and for a prolonged period of time, an energy disorder may start to affect a specific organ, or the excessive emotion might produce pathogenic fire in a specific organ.

In Western medicine and psychology, a dichotomy exists between body and mind, but this dichotomy does not exist in traditional Chinese medicine. Each internal organ is responsible for a specific emotion; conversely, each emotion acts on a specific internal organ. Thus, the heart gives rise to joy, the liver gives rise to anger, the lungs give rise to worry and sadness, the spleen gives rise to thought, the kidneys give rise to fear and shock. Conversely, joy mirrors and affects the state of the heart, anger mirrors and affects the state of the liver, worry and sadness mirror and affect the state of the lungs, thought mirrors and affects the state of the spleen, and fear and shock mirror and affect the state of the kidneys.

The *Nei Jing* says, "Anger is harmful to the liver, but sadness can reduce anger. Joy is harmful to the heart, but fear can reduce joy. Thought is harmful to the spleen, but anger can reduce thought. Worry and sadness are harmful to the lungs, but joy can reduce worry and sadness. Fear and shock are harmful to the kidneys, but thought can reduce fear." In effect, if you are suffering from an extreme emotion and thus causing disease to your body, it is advisable to summon up the balancing emotion. This viewpoint is supported by another Chinese medical classic, *Yi Lin Sheng,* published in 1584, which says, "Medicinal herbs alone cannot treat a disorder caused by an extreme emotion. Another emotion should be engaged to reduce the extreme emotion that is causing the disorder in order to strike a balance. . . . A healing emotion is an invisible herbal remedy."

In traditional Chinese medicine, one essential way to control emotions is to understand the relations among different emotions, that is, how emotions work on each other. Human emotions, like internal organs in the human body, are not isolated from each other; on the contrary, all emotions are related in three ways.

First, one emotion may give rise to another emotion, which in turn may give rise to yet another emotion. Anger gives rise to joy, joy gives rise to thought, thought gives rise to worry and sadness, worry and sadness give rise to fear and shock, fear and shock give rise to anger. Second, one emotion may overcome another emotion. Anger overcomes thought, thought overcomes fear and shock, fear and shock overcome joy, joy overcomes worry and sadness, and worry and sadness overcome anger. Third, one emotion may reduce the intensity of another emotion. Anger overcomes thought, but when excessive thought turns into fire, it reduces the intensity of anger, returning the body to a state of balance. Thought overcomes fear and shock, but when excessive fear and shock turn into fire, they reduce the intensity of thought. Fear and shock overcome joy, but when excessive joy turns into fire, it reduces fear and shock. Joy overcomes worry and sadness, but when excessive worry and sadness turn into fire, they reduce joy. Worry and sadness overcome anger, but when excessive anger turns into fire, it reduces worry and sadness.

Understanding the three ways in which emotions work on each other will help you control your emotions. If, for example, you feel you are constantly in a state of anger, which is harmful to your liver, you can increase your sadness to overcome your anger. This can be done, for example, by thinking about some sad scenes from a movie you have recently seen. If you feel very sad, which is harmful to your lungs, you can overcome your sadness by increasing your joy. You can do this by thinking about something that cheers you up. This method of controlling emotions is based on the theory I described above—that one emotion can overcome another emotion and that one emotion can increase or reduce the intensity of another emotion. The next time you feel angry with your spouse, remember that the more you feel angry with your partner, the more you love him or her, because anger can increase joy.

If you feel angry now, after your anger is gone you are very likely to be joyful, because anger gives rise to joy. If you feel joyful now, after your joy is gone, you are very likely to be in deep thought, because joy gives rise to thought. Throughout your life, you will have emotions that are constantly changing, from one to another according to the three basic patterns described above.

The following chart summarizes how you can control emotions to strike an emotional balance.

SEVEN EMOTIONS	HARMFUL TO CORRESPONDING ORGANS	MUTUAL REDUCTION
Joy	Excessive joy is harmful to the heart for two reasons. First, energy of the heart produces joy. Excessive joy consumes heart energy, which leads to deficient heart energy. Second, excessive joy relaxes the heart to the extent that the heart cannot focus on its activity, which impairs the capacity of the heart to function effectively.	1. Fear and shock overcome joy. It helps to eat more salty foods, which act on the kidney to reinforce fear and shock. 2. Worry and sadness reduce joy. It helps to eat more pungent foods, which act on the lungs to reinforce worry and sadness.
Anger	Excessive anger is harmful to the liver for two reasons. First, energy of the liver produces anger, and excessive anger consumes liver energy, which leads to deficient liver energy. Second, excessive anger makes liver energy rise up to the head, which may cause headache and impair the capacity of the liver to function effectively.	1. Worry and sadness overcome anger. It helps to eat more pungent foods, which act on the lung to reinforce worry and sadness. 2. Thought reduces anger. It helps to eat more sweet foods, which act on the spleen to reinforce thought.

SEVEN EMOTIONS	HARMFUL TO CORRESPONDING ORGANS	MUTUAL REDUCTION
Worry, sadness	Excessive worry and sadness are harmful to the lungs for two reasons. First, energy of the lungs produces worry and sadness, and excessive worry and sadness consume lung energy quickly, which leads to deficient lung energy. Second, excessive worry and sadness can cause abdominal pain and swelling and impair the capacity of the lungs to function effectively.	1. Joy overcomes worry and sadness. It helps to eat more bitter foods, which act on the heart to reinforce joy. 2. Anger reduces worry and sadness. It helps to eat more sour foods, which act on the liver to reinforce anger.
Thought	Excessive thought is harmful to the spleen for two reasons. First, energy of the spleen produces thought, and excessive thought consumes spleen energy, which leads to deficient spleen energy. Second, thought causes congestion of spleen energy, which impairs the capacity of the spleen to function effectively.	1. Anger overcomes thought. It helps to eat more sour foods, which act on the liver to produce the needed emotion of anger. 2. Fear and shock reduce the intensity of thought. It helps to eat more salty foods, which act on the kidneys to produce the needed emotions of fear and shock.
Fear, shock	Excessive fear and shock are harmful to the kidney for two reasons. First, energy of the kidneys produces fear and shock, and excessive fear and shock consume kidney energy, which leads to deficient kidney energy. Second, fear causes kidney energy to move downward, and shock causes a chaotic condition of kidney energy, both of which impair the capacity of the kidneys to function effectively.	1. Thought overcomes fear and shock. It helps to eat more sweet foods, which act on the spleen to reinforce thought. 2. Joy reduces fear and shock. It helps to eat more bitter foods to reinforce joy.

The following chart summarizes how to control your internal organs and emotions by eating certain foods.

EAT THE FOODS LISTED BELOW	TO ENHANCE THE ENERGY OF THE ORGANS	TO ENHANCE THE EMOTIONS	TO REDUCE THE EMOTIONS
Sour foods	Liver and gallbladder	Anger	Thought
Bitter foods	Heart and small intestine	Joy	Sadness and worry
Sweet foods	Spleen and stomach	Thought	Fear and shock
Pungent foods	Lungs and large intestine	Worry and sadness	Anger
Salty foods	Kidneys and bladder	Fear and shock	Joy

Foods and fatigue as mixed causes

FOODS

How do foods cause disease? We all know that specific foods or types of food can be bad for your health: sweet foods may cause diabetes, salt may cause hypertension, and saturated fats may cause heart disease. In traditional Chinese medicine, the role of foods is somewhat different. The way foods are eaten, the combinations of foods, and even eating habits may cause disease.

Irregular eating habits may cause disorders to the digestive system. The general rule is that you should eat only when hungry, drink only when thirsty, and stop eating when 80 percent full.

Eating the wrong foods under the wrong circumstances may cause diseases. When the body is in a particular state, certain foods may cause harm, particularly when you are ill. If you eat hot spicy foods such as cayenne pepper, cloves, and garlic while you have a high fever, a sore throat, constipation, or skin eruptions with red lesions, you are eating the wrong foods under the wrong circumstances, because such foods will intensify your symptoms.

Eating foods inconsistent with your physical constitution may also cause disease even though you are not really sick at the time. A specific food may be good for one physical constitution but bad for another, which means that the value of foods should be judged according to each individual's physical constitution (see Chapter 3).

FATIGUE

When you are ill, you may be advised to take it easy and rest for a few days, because the doctor believes your illness is due to fatigue. Western doctors in general are not very clear about exactly how fatigue causes disease or intensifies it, but doctors of traditional Chinese medicine are more specific about the relation between fatigue and disease.

There are five types of fatigue harmful to health: prolonged use of the eyes (excessive reading, watching television) is harmful to your blood; lying down for too long is harmful to your energy; prolonged sitting (at the computer, on a long airplane trip) is harmful to your muscles; prolonged standing is harmful to your bones, and prolonged walking is harmful to your tendons.

Excessive fatigue is particularly harmful to the spleen; it can cause a disease known as "spleen deficiency." Its symptoms include slightly cold hands and feet, abdominal swelling, skinniness or fatness with a poor appetite, chronic diarrhea, indigestion, the urge to lie down, morning sickness during pregnancy, excessive menstrual bleeding, irregular menstruation, anemia, and pale complexion.

Excessive sex also causes fatigue and it is particularly harmful to the kidneys, as it can cause a disease known as "kidney deficiency." Its symptoms are hair loss, frequent miscarriage and period pain in women, lower back pain, toothache, ringing in the ears, diabetes, heart palpitation, fear of cold, dizziness, short breath, cold feet, frequent urination, impotence in men and infertility in women, and cold sensations in the genitals.

CHAPTER 2

Meridians and Acupuncture

A chronic disease with a very long history can still be cured, and those
who think otherwise have not really mastered the art of acupuncture.
—NEI JING

What is Chinese acupuncture? Modern acupuncture is a therapeutic technique that involves the use of specially manufactured, extremely thin needles. These needles are inserted just beneath the skin at specific points on the body in order to stimulate the nerves for the purpose of curing diseases. These specific points are called acupuncture points, and the lines that connect the points are called meridians. Meridians are pathways along which energy travels through the body. There are a total of more than five hundred points and over fifty meridians, but a typical acupuncturist will use about one hundred points and engage fourteen major meridians.

Acupuncture dates back to ancient China. Chinese legend recounts that nine kinds of needles were manufactured for the treatment of diseases by Emperor Fu Xi (2852–2738 BC). Another legend relates that Chinese acupuncture began with the Yellow Emperor around 2698 BC. One thing is certain: the needles employed at the initial stage in the development of acupuncture treatment were made of stone, and for that reason it was recorded in Chinese medical classics that "the stones used to treat diseases were called stone-needles."

There are a number of major branches of traditional Chinese medicine, all of which are discussed in this book, but a TCM practitioner need not practice all the branches of TCM, although the vast majority of them do. Western health practitioners are particularly impressed by the effectiveness of acupuncture to relieve pain, which is indeed its most distinct feature.

Here is one story from my own practice. One day a patient called me to say that he had taken a terrible fall a few minutes earlier and was now in acute pain. He asked if I could relieve his pain with acupuncture.

"How many acupuncture treatments will I need?" he asked. "Anywhere from ten to twenty treatments," I replied. "Why do I need that many treatments? Can't you fix me by just one treatment?" I didn't know how to reply. He showed up about an hour later. We had to help him into the clinic from his car. I asked him to lie down on his stomach and started the treatment. Half an hour later, I finished the treatment and removed the needles in his body and told him to get up slowly. Once he was standing, he realized that the pain was completely gone.

Many years of special training are required to become an acupuncturist. The general descriptions given here should not be taken as a guide to practice acupuncture.

The theory of meridians

The development of the Chinese theory of meridians dates back to the Zhou dynasty (1122–255 BC). The *Nei Jing* describes in great detail the pathways of the meridians in the body and their therapeutic functions. However, the Chinese theory of meridians as a systematic theoretical framework did not come into existence all at once; it was gradually developed from three different kinds of experiences.

First of all, the ancient Chinese began to realize from their everyday experience that stimulation or pressure at a given point on the body may affect another region of the body; the stimulation transmits sensations along a line that travels between the two regions. Originally those points were stimulated manually, but needles are now more commonly used. When an acupuncture point is needled, the patient will feel sensations of soreness, distention, numbness, and heaviness radiating toward a fixed region of the body along a line, so to speak. The line along which the sensations radiate is called a meridian. As time went on, more and more lines were discovered—today, more than fifty meridians have been identified.

Second, the early Chinese acupuncturists, through their clinical experience, gradually learned that some categories of symptoms frequently occur simultaneously but are rarely observed in connection with other symptoms. These acupuncturists also observed that certain diseases often displayed the symptoms of pain, numbness, soreness, distention, and heaviness in a fixed region of the body. The Chinese acupuncturists gradually systematized their experiences and built the data gleaned from their observations into a logical theory in which the meridians are said to be connected with the internal organs. Because of this connection, the meridians are named after the organ's names—the stomach meridian, the large intestine meridian, the gallbladder meridian, and so forth.

Third, the Chinese people were in the habit of practicing Qi Gong, or energy exercises, which dates back to ancient China. When doing these exercises, they would concentrate on certain points of the body, and many of them noticed a stream of energy running through their whole body in a line. As an example, the stream of energy conventionally called "the small universe" that often circulates through the body in the midst of Qi Gong exercises is found to connect with areas known as the "governing meridian" in the back and the "conception meridian" in the front. The direct experience gathered from the exercises was applied to the theory of meridians.

The meridians in Chinese acupuncture are comparable to, but not identical to, the blood vessels or the nervous system in Western medicine. All in all, there are twelve master meridians, eight extraordinary meridians, twelve separate master meridians, twelve muscular meridians, and fifteen linking meridians. In addition, there are hundreds of other minor meridians in the human body that function like a network. The twelve master meridians are by far the most important and essential of all meridians in the human body.

The twelve master meridians in the human body run through the head, face, trunk, four extremities, and symmetrically through both sides of the body. Each master meridian is identified with an internal organ, and it is also linked with another organ. In addition, each master meridian travels through fixed regions on the body surface, and for that reason each is accessible for manipulation, making them particularly useful in the treatment of specific diseases.

Meridians circulate energy and blood to nourish and rejuvenate the whole body. The *Nei Jing* sums up the function of meridians, saying, "The meridians exist for the purpose of circulating blood and energy, rejuvenating yin and yang, moistening tendons and bones, as well as facilitating the functions of joints."

Acupuncture points and their relationship to meridians

Acupuncture points refer to the points on the body surface that connect with the meridians and the internal organs; they are the points at which the energy streams from the meridians spring up; they are also the points at which acupuncture and moxibustion treatment takes place. The literal meaning of the Chinese expression for acupuncture point contains two

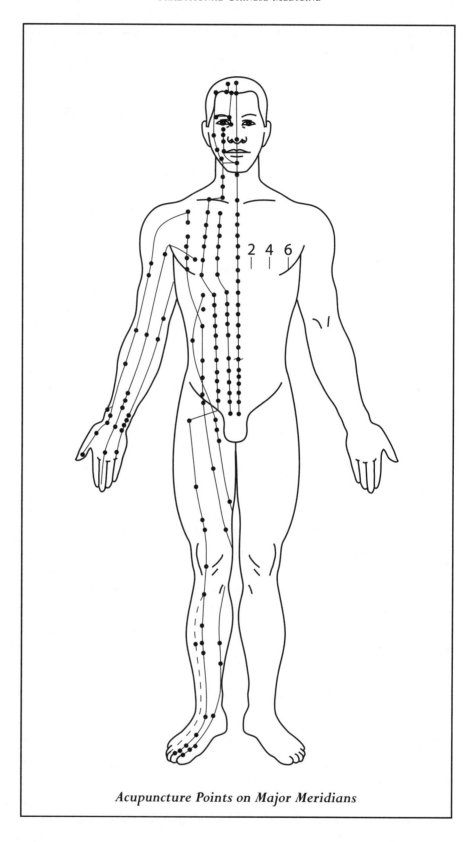

Acupuncture Points on Major Meridians

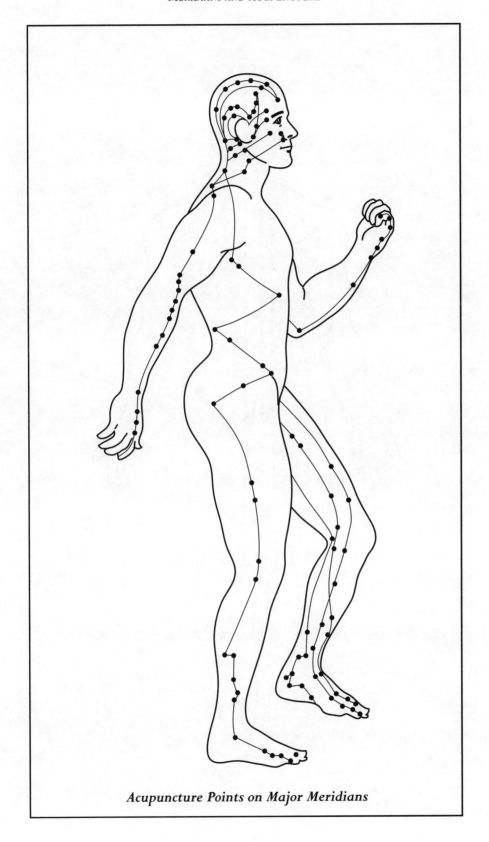

Acupuncture Points on Major Meridians

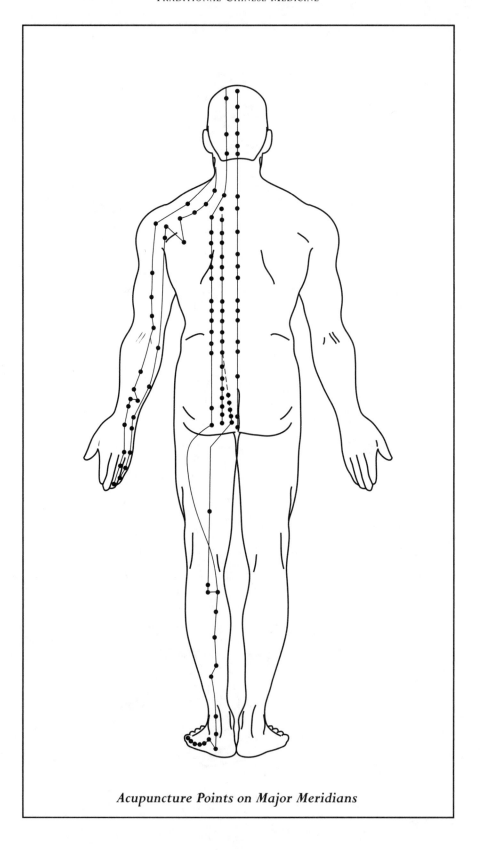

Acupuncture Points on Major Meridians

words, namely, *shu* and *xue*; *shu* means "flowing" and *xue* means "aperture." Therefore, the literal meaning of acupuncture point in the Chinese language is "flowing aperture," which means that acupuncture points are the stations through which energy streams flow or at which they gather. In Chinese, acupuncture points are also called "energy apertures" or "positions of apertures."

The places where acupuncture points are connected together or intersect are called "points of meridians." The points that are not on the meridians are called "extraordinary points outside the meridians" or simply "extraordinary points" or "extra points." In addition, tender points or pressure-painful points form the third category of acupuncture points. The *Nei Jing* advises, "The pressure-painful points may be taken as acupuncture points." Thus, acupuncture points contain three categories: the points of meridians, the extraordinary points, and the tender points, all of which are therapeutic points in acupuncture. The points on the fourteen major meridians are the most important ones, extraordinary points are supplemental points, and tender points are based on the affected regions, which are painful when pressure is applied. The fourteen major meridians refer to the twelve master meridians mentioned earlier, plus two other meridians—one traveling vertically through the central plane in the front called the "conception meridian" or *ren mai*, and the other through the central plane in the back called the "governing meridian" or *du mai*.

The practitioner of traditional Chinese medicine examines the body surface with a combination of visual observation and the application of pressure to various points. With these methods, it is possible to find many abnormal phenomena, such as disturbances of sensations, aching pain, tenderness, oversensitiveness, swelling, hardening, blood clotting, depression, and throbbing. The ancient Chinese applied various kinds of stimulations to such regions, including massage, pricking with a sharp stone, and warm moxibustion, all of which promote energy and blood circulation to alleviate pain. When energy and blood block or slow the circulation, it will cause all sorts of pain.

The practice of manipulating acupuncture points not only cures the diseases that occur in the local regions, but it can also cure diseases that are remote from the regions where the points are located. Acupuncture not only cures diseases on the body surface, but it also cures diseases in the body's cavities. Based on their observations and experiences, the ancient Chinese established the conception of meridians to connect the internal and the external, the local and remote regions of the human body. Such connections may be manifested through the radiating sensations felt by the patient during an acupuncture or moxibustion treatment—notably, the sensations of soreness, distension, heaviness, numbness, or heavy feelings felt in the acupuncturist's hands when inserting the needle, or radiating sensations of heat, all of which indicate the existence of energy streams at acupuncture points. Therefore, acupuncture points are referred to in the *Nei Jing* as "the points at which energy of meridians springs up." Thus, the physiological functions of acupuncture points are neither isolated nor chaotic or superficial, but rather they exist around the whole body and are connected with one another in a fixed and systematic pattern.

The *Nei Jing* presents a systematic summary of medical experience and theoretical knowledge as well as a thorough and comprehensive understanding of acupuncture points. The system of meridians, which are closely connected with acupuncture points, becomes one of the most important parts of this gigantic medical work, in which the guiding principles presented for clinical practice have gone beyond the concept of points and reached the concept of lines. Many acupuncture points belong to the same meridian, and the acupuncture points that belong to the same meridian are similar in their therapeutic functions.

Treatment functions of acupuncture points

The acupuncture points on the four extremities below the elbow and the knee are considered the fundamental points and form the basis for dividing meridians. This is why when you go to see a TCM doctor for acupuncture treatment, chances are the doctor will put needles in your four limbs, even though you may have a headache or a stomachache or perhaps a hearing problem—none of which occur in the four limbs.

Each meridian is identified by a letter or a syllable:
- *B* stands for the bladder meridian
- *D* stands for the Du or governing meridian
- *G* stands for the gallbladder meridian
- *H* stands for the heart meridian
- *K* stands for the kidney meridian
- *Li* stands for the large intestine meridian
- *Lu* stands for the lung meridian
- *Lv* stands for the liver meridian
- *P* stands for the pericardium meridian
- *R* stands for the Ren or conception meridian

S stands for the stomach meridian

Si stands for the small intestine meridian

Sj stands for the Sanjiao or "triple heater" meridian

Sp stands for the spleen meridian

All the points have a number. As an example, *K1* refers to the first point on the kidney meridian; *Li4* refers to the fourth point on the large intestine meridian. There are also Chinese names for each point; for example, *K1* is called "bubbling fountain."

Treatment of diseases using acupuncture points

Various other techniques use the acupuncture points: acupressure (shiatsu), moxibustion, and cupping.

ACUPRESSURE OR SHIATSU

Acupressure or shiatsu uses a variety of techniques to manipulate the same points as in acupuncture treatment. In many cases, acupressure is a fairly effective treatment. For example, in China, acupressure has been used as an anesthetic in dentistry. Three acupuncture points are pressed for just ten minutes before the teeth are pulled without pain or infection.

MOXIBUSTION

In moxibustion, dried mugwort leaves—either in a cigarlike stick or a paste—are lit and placed close to the acupuncture point to produce warm sensations. This method of treatment is most effective for the treatment of chronic diseases, such as indigestion, chronic diarrhea, stomachache, abdominal pain, period pain, and arthritis. However, moxibustion should not be applied to the face or used in the treatment of hot diseases. Nor is it applied to the abdominal region of a pregnant woman.

CUPPING

Cupping involves the use of a cup made of bamboo, earthenware, or glass to which heat is applied. Various sizes of cups are used on different regions of the body. A vacuum is created by burning a cotton ball in the cup, then quickly discarding the cotton and placing the cup firmly over the acupuncture point so that the cup attaches to the skin surface. The vacuum may last five to ten minutes, depending on the points engaged and the patient's comfort. You can also slide the attached cup back and forth on the skin to reinforce the effects.

Cupping is considered especially effective for the following symptoms: headache, dizziness, cough, pain, and swelling in the eyes—all due to the common cold. It is also effective for treating rheumatic pain, indigestion, abdominal pain, stomachache, and diarrhea.

Cupping should not be applied to skin diseases; in cases of sudden fainting, allergic reactions, or tumors; to the heart region, nipples, and the lower abdomen in pregnant women. If the patient feels uncomfortable or experiences burning pain, dizziness, nausea, or cold sweats, the cup should be removed immediately.

CHAPTER 3

Food and Herbal Cures

Medicinal herbs can attack diseases. Eat five grains for nourishment, eat five fruits and five vegetables as supplemental foods, and eat five domestic animals to benefit the body. —NEI JING

In traditional Chinese medicine many plants are considered both foods and herbs. In fact, there is a Chinese saying: "One cannot always draw a line between foods and herbs." Some herbs are so mild in effect and so pleasing to the taste that they can be eaten as food, such as Asian dandelion and Chinese yam; on the other hand, some foods contain powerful healing properties and are used as herbs, such as garlic and dried ginger. Because of the dual nature of so many foods and herbs, food cures have always been used side by side with herbal cures in China. That is, Chinese physicians often make it a point to advise their patients to take certain herbs and eat certain foods simultaneously in order to cure a disease.

Food Cures

The origins of food cures in traditional Chinese medicine date back to the Zhou dynasty (1122 BC–256 BC). During the Zhou, food cures were assigned to a department in the government alongside three other health departments—internal medicine, external medicine, and veterinary medicine. According to one count, more than three hundred classic works on food cures have been published in China since the Han dynasty (206 BC–AD 220), only sixteen of which are still in existence today.

The following is a list of symptoms and conditions and the foods used to treat them.

SYMPTOMS	FOOD CURES	SYMPTOMS	FOOD CURES
Abdominal obstruction	tofu	Alcoholism	freshwater clam
		Alcoholism, chronic	yam bean
Abdominal pain	buckwheat	Altitude sickness	fenugreek seed
	fennel seed		
	ginger, fresh	Anemia	corn silk
	green onion, white part only		longan
	hawthorn fruit	Angina pectoris	bee venom
	rosin		hawthorn fruit
	mutton or goat meat		
	sorghum	Appendicitis	purslane
	brown sugar		
	wild cabbage	Arrhythmia	chicken egg yolk
		Arsenic poisoning	eggplant
			radish leaf
		Arteriosclerosis	tea
			tofu
			eggplant
			wheat bran
			yam
		Arthritis	bee venom
			loquat root
			red vinespinach
			royal jelly
Abdominal pain with chills	grapefruit		sunflower disc or receptacle
	lichee		vinegar
	black pepper		
	red or green pepper (chili pepper, cayenne pepper)	Asthma	bamboo liquid oil
			black sesame seed
			cinnamon bark
Acute gastroenteritis	tea		cuttlebone
			squash
Aging	common button mushroom		grapefruit peel
	royal jelly		
	walnut		

Hawthorn fruit

SYMPTOMS	FOOD CURES	SYMPTOMS	FOOD CURES
Asthma, bronchial	castor bean pork testes bee venom	Blurred vision	liver (beef, chicken, pork) matrimony vine leaf
Bleeding	black fungus day lily white fungus lotus rhizome radish shepherd's purse water spinach	Breast cancer	crab squash calyx
		Breast lump	cucumber green onion (fibrous root) squash calyx
Bleeding after childbirth	lotus rhizome	Bronchitis	chicken jellyfish pork gallbladder tangerine peel water chestnut
Bleeding gums	white sugar		
Blocked urination	prickly ash		
Blood in stools	black sesame seed kumquat cake lichee longan mung bean sprouts chestnut eggplant kohlrabi leaf or brown mustard		
Blood in urine	celery lettuce towel gourd		

Jellyfish

Food cure for blood in urine with diminished urination

Cut up 50 g celery into small pieces. Place celery, 25 g broad beans, and 100 g rice in a saucepan and cover with water to about an inch above. Boil until soft. Eat at mealtime.

SYMPTOMS	FOOD CURES	SYMPTOMS	FOOD CURES
Bronchitis, chronic	fungus, white fungus yam	Colon cancer	Chinese chive
		Common cold	coriander (Chinese parsley) duck egg honeysuckle stem leaf pine leaf green onion, white part

Food cure for bronchitis
Rinse 100 g dried jellyfish. Place jellyfish and 100 g fresh chestnuts in a saucepan and cover with water to about an inch above. Boil until soft. Eat at mealtime, once a day, until the symptoms disappear.

Food cure for the common cold
Combine 6 green onions, white part only, 50 g maltose (or brown sugar if not available), and 2 cups (500 mL) water. Bring to a boil for a few seconds. Discard the onions. Add an egg white into the soup and stir. Divide into three doses to drink morning, afternoon, and evening.

SYMPTOMS	FOOD CURES	SYMPTOMS	FOOD CURES
Burn	cucumber mung bean mung bean powder pork skin watermelon		
Cancer	apricot button mushroom carrot Chinese gooseberry eggplant leaf garlic lily bulb leaf ling mulberry root bark snail (river snail) wild cabbage	Concussion	peanut plant
		Conjunctivitis	peanut oil pork gallbladder
		Constipation	bamboo shoot black sesame seed carrots green onion, white part loquat leaf
Canker, mouth	watermelon		
Cardiovascular diseases	Chinese chive	Constipation	potato red vinespinach small white cabbage sweet potato water spinach
Cervical cancer	shiitake mushroom walnut twig (young branches)		
Chickenpox	potato		
Childbirth, difficult	pork		
Cirrhosis	azuki bean		

Food cure for constipation
Cut 250 g carrots into cubes. Boil in water until soft. Eat at mealtime.

SYMPTOMS	FOOD CURES	SYMPTOMS	FOOD CURES
Constipation in the elderly	walnut	Cough	betel pepper
			citron
			crown daisy
Constipation with dry stools	amaranth		goose meat
	banana		mandarin orange
	beef		olive
	black sesame seed		peanut
	carrot		pear
	fungus, white fungus		squash
	honey		
	longevity fruit	Cough, chronic	chicken
	mulberry		lily bulb leaf
	peach		
	pine-nut kernel	Cough (dry cough)	apple
	pork		autumn bottle gourd
	spinach		banana
			fungus, white fungus
			honey
			peanut
			pine-nut kernel
			pork
			sand pear
			sugar cane

Food cure for constipation with dry stools
Boil 100 g spinach in water until soft. Drain. Pour 1 teaspoon sesame oil over the spinach. Eat at mealtime.

SYMPTOMS	FOOD CURES	SYMPTOMS	FOOD CURES
Corns	yellow soybean sprout		
		Cough due to weak lungs	plum (prunes)
Coronary heart disease	tofu		
	black fungus	Cough with chills	leaf or brown mustard
	chrysanthemum		
	hawthorn fruit	Cough with copious phlegm	apricot
			bamboo shoot
			chicken egg
			ginkgo (cooked)
			grapefruit
			towel gourd
			water chestnut

Food cure for coronary heart disease
Immerse 6 g black fungus in water for 20 minutes. Cut up 50 g lean pork. Combine the pork and the black fungus with 30 g cornstarch and add to 2 cups (500 mL) water. Boil to make soup. Eat the soup at mealtime, once a day.

SYMPTOMS	FOOD CURES
Coughing up blood	duck
	loquat
	persimmon

Food cure for coronary heart disease with hypertension
Place 50 g cornstarch, 10 g rice, and 10 g of tofu in a saucepan. Cover with water to about an inch above. Boil to make soup. Eat at mealtime, once a day.

SYMPTOMS	FOOD CURES	SYMPTOMS	FOOD CURES
Cystitis	magnolia vine fruit, Chinese red vinespinach	Diabetes (continued)	wheat bran winter melon yam
Decreased vision	matrimony vine leaf		
Dehydration	coconut meat		
Depression	red date wheat		
Dermatitis	chicken egg pork gallbladder rice bran oil safflower tea walnut walnut twig (young branches)	Diarrhea	black pepper brown sugar buckwheat sprout chestnut chicken garlic
Diabetes	bottle gourd black fungus corn (sweet or Indian) eggplant hyacinth bean kiwi fruit mulberry palm seed pear pork pancreas radish sand pear sheep or goat's pancreas spinach squash sweet potato vine leaves tangerine orange water spinach		grapefruit leaf hyacinth bean onion papaya purslane rabbit liver red bayberries

Food cure for diabetes
Cut 150 g squash and 100 g yam into small pieces. Place in a saucepan and cover with water to about an inch above. Eat the soup at mealtime.

Chestnut

Food cure for diarrhea
Place 30 g hyacinth beans and 100 g rice in a saucepan. Cover with water to about an inch above. Eat at mealtime.

SYMPTOMS	FOOD CURES	SYMPTOMS	FOOD CURES
Diarrhea (continued)	tangerine orange watermelon yam	Diminished urination (continued)	cucumber grapes green onion, white part hami melon kidney bean lettuce mandarin orange mango mulberry red vinespinach star fruit string bean winter melon
Diarrhea, chronic	apple carrot fig gorgan fruit guava lichee lotus rhizome plum (prunes) pomegranate (sweet fruit) sword bean wheat		
		Diphtheria	pork gallbladder walnut
		Dizziness	corn silk
		Dog bite	apricot seed (bitter)
		Dry eyes	liver (pork)
Diarrhea, with indigestion	pineapple	Dry throat	apricot
Diarrhea in infant	tea	Dysentery	amaranth bitter gourd (balsam pear) cantaloupe chicken gall bladder Chinese toon leaf chrysanthemum cucumber vine (stem) date tree bark fig garlic ginger, fresh grape guava
Digestive tract disorders	black fungus		
Diminished urination	amaranth asparagus barley bottle gourd cantaloupe carp celery Chinese cabbage crown daisy		

Food cure for chronic diarrhea
Peel 2 apples. Remove the seeds. Cut up and place in a saucepan. Cover with water to about an inch above. Boil until soft. Drink the liquid like tea.

SYMPTOMS	FOOD CURES	SYMPTOMS	FOOD CURES

Dysentery (continued)	hawthorn fruit
	honeysuckle
	hyacinth bean flower
	lotus root
	magnolia vine fruit,
	  Chinese
	olive
	papaya
	plum (prunes)
	pomegranate (sweet
	  fruit and peel)
	purslane
	radish leaf
	red vinespinach
	scallion bulb
	smoked prunes
	tea
	tomato
	towel gourd
	walnut leaf
		Edema (continued)	beef
			bottle gourd
			carp (common and
			  gold)
			chicken
			corn (Indian corn,
			  maize)
			day lily
			duck
			grapes
			kidney bean
			kohlrabi
			mulberry
			radish leaf
			shepherd's purse
			sorghum root
			winter melon

Food cure for dysentery
Cut up a garlic clove into five pieces and crush them. Divide into two equal doses. Wash down one dose with warm water, twice daily.

Food cure for edema
Cut 50 g winter melon into cubes. Place melon and 50 g kidney beans in a saucepan. Cover with water to about an inch above. Boil until soft. Eat at mealtime.

SYMPTOMS	FOOD CURES	SYMPTOMS	FOOD CURES

Earache
  (Otitis media)
	pork gallbladder	Edema during
		  pregnancy
			carp

Eczema	broad bean shell chicken egg yolk clam, freshwater coconut shell mung bean powder olive potato soybean, black	Encephalitis	banana rhizome buffalo's horn pine leaf
		Enteritis	chicken egg Chinese toon leaf date tree bark ginkgo (cooked) kumquat pork gallbladder purslane tea
Edema	areca nuts autumn bottle gourd		

SYMPTOMS	FOOD CURES	SYMPTOMS	FOOD CURES
Epilepsy	castor bean root green turtle olive	Genital itch	apricot seed (bitter) chicken egg yolk
		Glaucoma	areca nuts
Fatigue	beef goose meat honey	Goiter	kelp laver
Fatigue, chronic	matrimony vine fruit mutton		
Food poisoning	ginger, fresh		
Forgetfulness	longan	Headache	buckwheat carp radish

Fracture	chicken egg shell inner
	    membrane
	mung bean powder
		Headache with the
		common cold
			green onion, white
			    part

Frostbite	cherry cherry juice chili rhizome rosin tangerine orange peel	Heart disease	ginkgo leaf hawthorn fruit loquat seed pineapple tea plant root
Fungus infections	bee secretion	Hemophilia	lotus rhizome peanut
Gallstone	radish		
Gastroduodenal ulcer	barley green peel of unripe walnut honey potato royal jelly	Hemorrhoid	black fungus clam, freshwater egg, chicken eggplant fig leaf or brown mustard pork
Gastric ulcer	wild cabbage		pork gallbladder spinach
Gastritis	papaya rice (polished)		walnut leaf water spinach

Food cure for goiter
Place 50 g kelp and 50 g laver in a saucepan. Cover with water to about an inch above. Boil until soft. Eat at mealtime.

SYMPTOMS	FOOD CURES	SYMPTOMS	FOOD CURES
Hemorrhoid (continued)	fig leaf	Hiccups triggered by cold	lichee
Hepatitis	button mushroom		
	cotton root	High cholesterol	celery
	garlic		corn (Indian corn, maize)
	glutinous rice stalk		cucumber
	honeysuckle stem leaf		garlic
	loach		kiwi fruit
	loquat root		onion
	magnolia vine fruit, Chinese		shiitake mushroom
	malt		sunflower seed
	muskmelon calyx receptacle		tofu
	pork gallbladder	Hookworm	purslane
	red and black date		
	rice straw	Hot sensations	pear
	royal jelly		
	tea	Hyperglycemia	black sesame seed
			water spinach
Hernia	green onion (white part, outer skin)		
		Hypersensitive dentin	tea
	pork		
		Hypertension	apple
Herpes	purslane		betel pepper
	water spinach		black sesame seed
			broad bean flower
Hiccups	brown sugar		carrot
	Chinese chive seeds		celery
	duck egg		chrysanthemum
	ginger, fresh		corn (Indian corn, maize)
	persimmon calyx receptacle		cucumber vine (stem)
	rice (polished rice)		eggplant
	sword bean and seed		garlic
			hawthorn fruit
			jellyfish
			matrimony vine root bark
			onion

Food cure for hiccups
Grind 10 dried lichee nuts (shells removed) into a fine powder. Mix the powder in 1 cup (250 mL) water with 2 tablespoons of brown sugar. Drink it as a tea.

SYMPTOMS	FOOD CURES	SYMPTOMS	FOOD CURES
Hypertension (continued)	peanut peanut plant peony rootbark	Hypothyroidism	kelp laver
		Hysteria	wheat
		Impotence	Chinese chive lobster mutton walnut

	persimmon
	persimmon calyx
	  receptacle
	royal jelly
	sand pear
	seaweed
	spinach
	sunflower disc or
	  receptacle
	sunflower leaf
	tofu
	tomato
	watermelon
		Indigestion	apricot seed (bitter)
			chicken egg yolk
			coriander, Chinese
			  parsley
			corncob
			grapefruit
			hawthorn fruit
			lemon
			papaya
			pomegranate leaf
			prickly ash
			sorghum
			tea
			water chestnut

		Indigestion in children	coconut meat

		Induced labor	asparagus (lucid
			  asparagus)
			sweet potato vine
			  leaves

Hyperthyroidism	persimmon	Infertility	ginger, fresh
		Inflammatory disease	chili pepper (cayenne pepper)
		Influenza	garlic

Food cure for hypertension with high cholesterol
Crush 250 g fresh celery to make celery juice. Drink in 1 day.

Food cure for hypertension with heart disease
Immerse 50 g hawthorn fruit in water for 15 minutes. Remove the fruit from the water and squeeze to obtain juice. Boil the juice over low heat to increase its concentration. Mix it with 50 g rice to make soup. Drink the soup at mealtime.

Food cure for hyperthyroidism
Crush 1 kg unripe persimmons. Fry until soft. Add 3 teaspoons honey and continue to fry until very sticky. Take 1 teaspoon 3 times a day.

SYMPTOMS	FOOD CURES	SYMPTOMS	FOOD CURES
Injury	chili pepper (cayenne pepper) glutinous rice stalk safflower	Intoxication	mandarin orange peanut sand pear tea tea melon
Lactation problems	carp button mushroom day lily fig lettuce papaya towel gourd	Itch	mung bean powder
		Jaundice	autumn bottle gourd brown sugar citron leaf corn male flower crab eggplant hawthorn fruit jackfruit kiwi fruit
Insomnia	lotus (fruit, seed, root) grapes lily bulb leaf longan peanut plant		

Food cure for insomnia
Place 15 longan nuts, 7 red dates, and 50 g rice in a saucepan. Cover with water to about an inch above. Boil until soft. Eat at mealtime.

Food cure for jaundice
Cut 50 g eggplant into cubes. Place eggplant, 100 g rice and 5 pieces ginger in a saucepan. Cover with water to about an inch above. Boil until soft. Eat at mealtime.

SYMPTOMS	FOOD CURES	SYMPTOMS	FOOD CURES
Intestinal obstruction	brown sugar ginger, fresh green onion, white part peanut oil prickly ash radish rapeseed (canola) oil soybean oil tea oil	Kidney disease	hami melon watermelon
		Laryngitis	watermelon
Intestinal parasites	areca nuts	Lead poisoning	mung bean water chestnut
Intoxication	apple grapefruit ling		

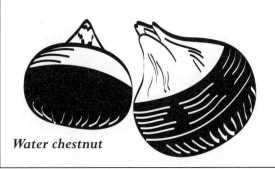

Water chestnut

SYMPTOMS	FOOD CURES	SYMPTOMS	FOOD CURES
Leukemia	hairtail	Meningitis	garlic
Loss of voice	fig longevity fruit loquat mango radish	Menorrhagia	sorghum root
		Menstrual cramps	hawthorn fruit lichee seed
		Menstruation, irregular	brown sugar ginger, fresh safflower
Malaria	areca nuts black pepper chicken egg		
		Migraine	muskmelon calyx receptacle radish
Malnutrition	squash		

Mastitis	chicken egg yolk
	eggplant
	grapevine leaf
	green onion, white
	  part
	honeycomb, wax cells
	kumquat seed
	pomegranate peel
	sunflower disc or
	  receptacle
	tangerine orange peel,
	  seed
		Miscarriage	azuki bean sprout

		Motion sickness	mango
		Mumps	black pepper mung bean potato
		Nervousness	longan wheat
		Neurosis	red date
Mastitis, acute	antler (deerhorn)	Night blindness	alfalfa root carrot liver (beef, chicken, pork) alfalfa root matrimony vine leaf spinach
Measles	shepherd's purse towel gourd		
Measles, early stage	cherry		

Measles, delayed
  eruption
	bamboo shoot
	coriander, Chinese
	  parsley
	shiitake mushroom
	sugar cane
		Night sweats	duck
			grapes

Food cure for night sweats
Peel and cut up 10 g yam. Place yam, 50 g rock sugar and 50 g rice in a saucepan. Cover with water to about an inch above. Eat at mealtime.

SYMPTOMS	FOOD CURES	SYMPTOMS	FOOD CURES
Night sweats (continued)	oyster shell peach rock sugar		
Nipple, sore	clove		
Nosebleed	chestnut Chinese chive green onion leaf radish spinach vinegar		
Numbness	black fungus		
Numbness of four limbs	cherry		
Obesity	winter melon yam		

Food cure for palpitations
Place 50 g longan nuts, 10 g lotus fruit and seed, and 50 g rice in a saucepan. Cover with water to about an inch above. Boil the three ingredients until soft. Eat at mealtimes.

SYMPTOMS	FOOD CURES
Penis swelling	green onion leaf
Peptic ulcer	banana wild cabbage
Periodontal disease	bee secretion
Perspiration	radish
Pink eye (conjunctivitis)	chicken egg cucumber shepherd's purse
Pneumonia	garlic honeysuckle (dried) jackfruit

Food cure for obesity
Boil 250 g winter melon in 3 cups (750 mL) water until soft. Eat the soup as a daily tonic.

Food cure for pneumonia
Prepare an infusion of 30 g dried honeysuckle and 6 g peppermint to make tea. Drink the tea at mealtimes.

SYMPTOMS	FOOD CURES	SYMPTOMS	FOOD CURES
Osteoporosis	chestnut		
Pain in the arm	carp (gold carp)		
Pain in the leg	chili pepper (cayenne pepper)	Poor appetite	black pepper cantaloupe honey kiwi fruit onion shiitake mushroom tangerine orange tomato
Pain in penis	sunflower root		
Pain in the testes	kumquat seed		
Pain in the tongue	bee venom		
Palpitations	grapes longan	Poor memory	tofu

SYMPTOMS	FOOD CURES	SYMPTOMS	FOOD CURES
Postnatal	icken	Sinusitis	peanut
	gus	Skin disease	castor bean
	chive	Skin inflammation	green onion, white part
	it, seed,	Sore throat	chicken egg cucumber fig longevity fruit olive radish star fruit
	gg runes		
	oked) mutton	Stomach cancer	Chinese chive shiitake mushroom sunflower stem and pith walnut twig (young branches) wild cabbage
Rheumatoid arthritis	bee venom chili pepper (cayenne pepper) royal jelly		
Rhinitis	aloe vera garlic magnolia flower bud peony rootbark sesame oil sword bean seed		
Ringing in the ears	day lily		
Scarlet fever	burdock garlic		
Scrotom swelling	lichee seed		
Seminal emission	duck gorgan fruit string bean yam		

Shiitake mushrooms

SYMPTOMS	FOOD CURES	SYMPTOMS	FOOD CURES
Stomachache	green peel of unripe walnut longan papaya potato sorghum leaf, root	Thirst (continued) Thrush	red bayberries sand pear star fruit tomato sesame oil
Stomachache with chills	garlic ginger, fresh grapefruit lichee	Thyroid cyst Toothache	seaweed olive prickly ash star fruit wax cells of honeycomb
Sunstroke	bitter gourd (balsam pear) hyacinth bean		
Swallowing difficulty	Chinese chive	Tuberculosis	chicken egg yolk garlic ginkgo (fresh or cooked) honeysuckle rabbit radish seaweed sheep or goat's gall bladder
Swollen scrotum	garlic		
Swollen testes	kelp		
Tetanus	green onion, white part mulberry branch juices		
Thirst	apple apricot bitter gourd (balsam pear) kiwi fruit lemon loquat mandarin orange olive pear pineapple plum (prunes) pomegranate (sweet fruit)	Tumors Tympanic membrane perforation Ulcer	asparagus (lucid asparagus) sunflower disc or receptacle kidney bean sword bean seed ginger, dried chicken egg shell inner membrane clam shell powder cuttlebone

SYMPTOMS	FOOD CURES	SYMPTOMS	FOOD CURES
Ulcer (continued)	ginger, fresh mung bean onion peanut oil potato safflower soybean, yellow	Vaginitis	Chinese toon leaf
		Vertigo	celery day lily liver, beef mulberry shepherd's purse
Urinary infection	watermelon	Vomiting	ginger, fresh loquat
Urination difficulty	arrowhead autumn bottle gourd garlic kohlrabi pear white cabbage wheat		lotus sprout mango red bayberries sugar cane sword bean and seed tangerine orange

Food cure for vomiting
Cut up fresh ginger into five pieces. Boil in water. Drink like tea.

SYMPTOMS	FOOD CURES	SYMPTOMS	FOOD CURES
Urination, frequent	gorgan fruit lotus (fruit, seed, root) mutton	Wart	yellow soybean sprout

Vaginal bleeding	asparagus (lucid
	  asparagus)
	cuttlefish ink sac
	persimmon cake
	sunflower disc or
	  receptacle
		Whooping cough	aloe vera
			asparagus
			chestnut
			chicken egg yolk
			purslane
			celery

Vaginal bleeding and discharge	chicken		chicken egg chicken gall bladder cow's gall bladder
Vaginal bleeding during pregnancy	liver, chicken		garlic longevity fruit pork gallbladder
Vaginal discharge	cuttlefish ginkgo (cooked)		sweet orange peel tofu

Herbal Cures

In traditional Chinese medicine, the distinction between foods and herbs is not hard and fast. For example, almonds, garlic, ginger, and green onions are all common food but they are also important herbs. However, there are two fundamental differences between herbs and foods. For one thing, many herbs do not taste good. When we are sick, we eat herbs in spite of their awful taste in order to get better. In the second place, herbs are stronger than foods in their therapeutic effects. Herbal cures can speed recovery faster than food cures, and in the case of a severe disease, herbs can do a much better job in facilitating recovery. For example, with food cures, a common cold will improve in three to four days, but by taking herbs recovery will occur within one or two days.

In the process of finding foods, our ancestors must have mistakenly eaten poisonous foods from time to time, which caused vomiting, diarrhea, or even death. From such experiences, they gradually came to identify which plants were edible and which were poisonous but could be used to heal disease.

DISEASE	SYMPTOMS AND SIGNS	HERBAL FORMULAS
Abdominal pain	acute, with chills, poor appetite, no thirst	Ling-Fu-Tang
	chronic, improves with heat, with soft stools	Xiao-Jian-Zhong-Tang
	with thirst, perspiration, and constipation, worsens with massage	Da-Cheng-Qi-Tang
	migratory pain that may extend to the chest or lower abdomen, improves on belching but worsens with emotional upset	Si-Ni-San
	pain in fixed spot, worsens with massage	Shao-Fu-Zhu-Yu-Tang
	worsens with massage, improves after bowel movement, with belching and acid reflux	Bao-He-Wan
Asthma	no thirst, thin, white phlegm	Ma-Huang-Tang
	thirst, yellowish phlegm	Ma-Xing-Shi-Gan-Tang
	with insomnia or chest congestion and pain	Wu-Mo-Yin-Zi
	with low voice and aversion to wind	Bu-Fei-Tang
	with urination disorders	Ren-Shen-Hu-Tao-Tang
	with wheezing and chills	She-Gan-Ma-Huang-Tang
	with wheezing and fever or hot sensations	Ding-Chuan-Tang

DISEASE	SYMPTOMS AND SIGNS	HERBAL FORMULAS
Bleeding gums	with swollen gums, bad breath, headache, constipation, red tongue with light-red, puffy gums, loose teeth, mild toothache, or dizziness and vertigo, ringing in the ears, lumbago, reddish tongue	Qing-Wei-San Zi-Shui-Qing-Gan-Yin
Blood in stools	red blood in stools, or discharge of blood before bowel movement, watery stools or abdominal pain discharge of blood in dark purple or black stools, or discharge of blood after bowel movement, or blood and stools mixed together, mild abdominal pain, love of warmth and massage, watery stools, fatigue, pale complexion, pale tongue	Chi-Xiao-Dou-Dang-Gui-San Huang-Tu-Tang
Blood in urine	burning sensation on urination, red blood in urine, insomnia, dry throat with thirst, red tongue blood in urine, dizziness, ringing in the ears, reddish cheeks, lumbago, reddish tongue light red blood in urine for a prolonged period, particularly when fatigued, lumbago, poor appetite, dizziness, ringing in the ears, pale tongue	Xiao-Ji-Yin-Zi Zhi-Bai-Di-Huang-Wan Gui-Pi-Tang

DISEASE	SYMPTOMS AND SIGNS	HERBAL FORMULAS
Chest pain on the side of the chest	migratory pain that worsens on emotional upset, with frequent belching and poor appetite	Chai-Hu-Shu-Gan-San
	pricking pain in fixed spot, worsens with massage, more severe at night	Xuan-Fu-Hua-Tang
	with nausea and vomiting, alternating chills and fever, yellowish appearance, yellowish or reddish urine	Long-Dan-Xie-Gan-Tang
	mild but constant pain, dry mouth and dry throat, mental depression, insomnia, dizziness, reddish tongue	Yi-Guan-Jian

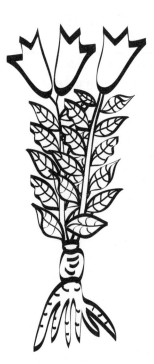

Long-dan (radix gentianae)
The key ingredient in Long-Dan-Xie-Gan-Tang, an herbal formula effective in treating chest pain on the side of the chest, deafness, ringing in the ears, eye disease, headache, herpes, hypertension, impotence, infections, nosebleed, and vomiting of blood.

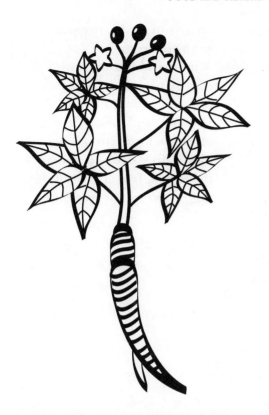

Ren-shen (radix ginseng)
The key ingredient in Si-Jun-Zi-Tang, an herbal formula effective in treating gastrointestinal disorders, poor appetite, and chronic fatigue.

DISEASE	SYMPTOMS AND SIGNS	HERBAL FORMULAS
Chronic fatigue	poor appetite, watery stools, excessive perspiration, palpitations, shortness of breath, frequent urination	Si-Jun-Zi-Tang
	palpitations, many dreams, forgetfulness, dizziness, mild chest pain, ringing in the ears, pale tongue	Gui-Pi-Tang
	underweight, watery stools, poor digestion, cold limbs, chills, diminished urination, pale tongue	You-Gui-Wan
	dry throat, dry cough, thirst with craving for drink, underweight, dry skin, constipation, night sweats, reddish tongue	Sha-Shen-Mai-Dong-Tang
Common cold	with chills	Jing-Fang-Bai-Du-San
	with fever	Yin-Qiao-San
	with dry cough, particularly in autumn	Sang-Xing-Tang
	with hot sensations, particularly in summer	Xin-Jia-Xiang-Ru-San

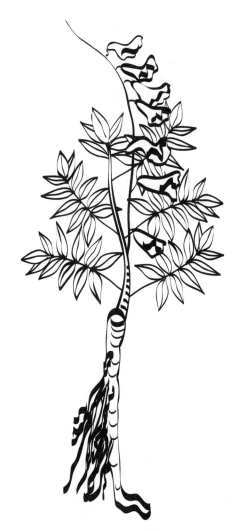

Huang-qi (radix astragali seu hedysari)
A mild and harmonious energy tonic, and a key ingredient in Bu-Zhong-Yi-Qi-Tang, an herbal formula effective in treating low blood pressure and urinary disorders. It is also used during recovery after an injury.

DISEASE	SYMPTOMS AND SIGNS	HERBAL FORMULAS
Constipation	with abdominal swelling, bad breath, dry mouth, reddish urine	Ma-Zi-Ren-Wan
	constant desire to empty the bowels without success, belching, abdominal pain, poor appetite	Liu-Mo-Tang
	accompanied by forgetfulness, palpitations, dizziness	Run-Chang-Wan
	constant desire to empty the bowels without success, fatigue after bowel movement	Huang-Qi-Tang
	difficult bowel movement with chills and abdominal pain, clear urine	Ji-Chuan-Jian

DISEASE	SYMPTOMS AND SIGNS	HERBAL FORMULAS
Cough	with chills with fever dry cough with copious phlegm weak cough	Zhi-Sou-San Sang-Ju-Yin Sang-Xing-Tang Er-Chen-Tang Bu-Fei-Tang
Coughing up blood	blood in phlegm, itchy, dry throat, reddish tongue blood in phlegm, pain induced by coughing, prone to anger, bitter taste in the mouth, reddish tongue scanty phlegm containing blood or coughing up blood in red, dry throat, red cheeks, night sweats, reddish tongue	San-Xing-Tang Xie-Bai-San Bai-He-Gu-Jin-Tang
Deafness, ringing in the ears	sudden onset, headache, reddish complexion, bitter taste in mouth, prone to anger ringing like the noise of a cicada, occasional blockage of the ear to cause total loss of hearing, copious phlegm, bitter taste in the mouth sudden ringing with loss of hearing, fever and headache, vomiting, itch inside the ears, sore throat dizziness and vertigo, seminal emission, reddish tongue, pain in lower back ringing and deafness with fatigue, palpitations, shortness of breath, dizziness and vertigo, watery stools	Long-Dan-Xie-Gan-Tang Wen-Dan-Tang Yin-Qiao-San Er-Long-Zuo-Zi-Wan Yi-Qi-Cong-Ming-Tang

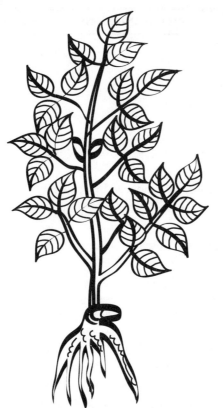

Huo-xiang (herba agastachis)
The key ingredient in Huo-Xiang-Zheng-Qi-San, an herbal formula effective in treating diarrhea, acute gastroenteritis, and vomiting.

DISEASE	SYMPTOMS AND SIGNS	HERBAL FORMULAS
Diarrhea	watery stools, abdominal pain and rumbling, chills or fever, poor appetite, headache and nasal congestion	Huo-Xiang-Zheng-Qi-San
	with urgent desire to empty the bowels, offensive smell, burning sensations in the anus, thirst	Ge-Gen-Qin-Lian-Tang
	with indigestion, offensive smell, pain improves after bowel movement	Bao-He-Wan
	with abdominal pain often triggered by emotional upset, with belching and poor appetite	Tong-Xie-Yao-Fang
	with indigestion that comes and goes, feeling of discomfort after bowel movement, fatigue	Shen-Ling-Bai-Zhu-San
	normally occurs before dawn, with abdominal pain surrounding the navel, abdominal rumbling preceding diarrhea, chills with cold limbs	Si-Shen-Wan

DISEASE	SYMPTOMS AND SIGNS	HERBAL FORMULAS
Edema	puffy eyelids gradually extending to the whole body, rapid progression, heavy sensations in the limbs and joints, diminished urination, aversion to cold and wind, fever	Yue-Bi-Jia-Zhu-Tang
	puffy eyelids gradually extending to the whole body, skin problems, aversion to wind, fever, reddish tongue	Ma-Huang-Lian-Qiao-Chi-Xiao-Dou-Tang
	puffy limbs, deep depressions from finger pressure, feeling of heaviness in the body, nausea, pale tongue	Wu-Ling-San
	puffiness in the whole body, shiny appearance of the skin, thirst, reddish urine, constipation with dry stools	Shu-Zao-Yin-Zi
	puffiness below the waist, depression caused by finger pressure rebounds to its original contours slowly when pressure is released	Shi-Pi-Yin
	puffy face with swollen body particularly below the waist, depression caused by finger pressure fails to rebound to its original contours when pressure is released, lumbago, decreased urination, cold limbs	Zhen-Wu-Tang
Headache	constant, affecting the back of neck that gets worse on windy days, chills, fatigued limbs, no thirst	Chuan-Xiong-Cha-Tiao-San
	with swelling sensations, severe headache as if the head about to burst, thirst, cough, sore throat	Sang-Ju-Yin
	as if the head wrapped up with a wet towel, diminished urination, watery stools, heavy sensations in the body	Qiang-Huo-Sheng-Shi-Tang
	with dizziness, prone to anger, poor sleep	Tian-Ma-Gou-Teng-Yin
	as if the head were empty inside, ringing in the ears, reddish tongue	Da-Bu-Yuan-Jian
	chronic, with intermittent occurrences, worse with fatigue, chills, poor appetite	Shun-Qi-He-Zhong-Tang
	with dizziness, dry eyes, poor complexion, palpitations, poor sleep, pale tongue	Jia-Wei-Si-Wu-Tang
	history of traumatic injury to the head, headache in a fixed spot	Tong-Qiao-Huo-Xue-Tang

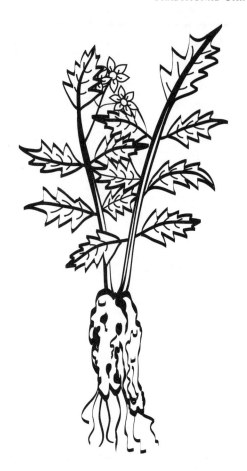

Dang-gui (radix angelicae sinensis)
A key ingredient in Si-Wu-Tang, an herbal formula effective in treating dizziness, impaired hearing, itchy skin, irregular menstruation, and vision impairment after an injury.

DISEASE	SYMPTOMS AND SIGNS	HERBAL FORMULAS
Heart pain	sudden, severe pain that worsens with cold, with chills and shortness of breath, affecting the back in severe cases	Dang-Gui-Si-Ni-Tang
	choking chest pain that affects the shoulder and the back, with cough, fatigue and abdominal swelling	Gua-Lou-Xie-Bai-Ban-Xia-Tang
	pain in a fixed spot as if cut by a knife, occasionally affecting the shoulder and the back	Xue-Fe-Zhu-Yu-Tang
	with dizziness, palpitations, fatigue, and pale complexion	Ba-Zhen-Tang
	intermittent, with palpitations and fatigue, insomnia, dry mouth and throat, constipation with dry stools, night sweats, tooth marks on the sides of tongue	Tian-Wang-Bu-Xin-Dan
	with shortness of breath and palpitations, chills and cold limbs, fatigue and pale complexion	Shen-Fu-Tang

DISEASE	SYMPTOMS AND SIGNS	HERBAL FORMULAS
Hiccups	occurring mostly in cold environments with poor appetite	Ding-Xiang-San
	high-pitched hiccup with bad breath or thirst and constipation	Zhu-Ye-Zhu-Ru-Tang
	triggered by emotional upset, chest discomfort and poor appetite	Wu-Mo-Yin-Zi
	with intermittent and low sound, fatigue, poor appetite, and cold limbs	Li-Zhong-Tang
	with quick but intermittent sound, dry throat and thirst	Yi-Wei-Tang
Impotence	dizziness, poor spirits, pain in lower back, pale tongue	Zan-Yu-Dan
	palpitations, timid, pale complexion, poor appetite, pale tongue	Da-Bu-Yin-Wan
	mental depression, chest discomfort, or discomfort in the lower abdomen	Xiao-Yao-San
	reddish urine or dribbling after urination, weakness of lower limbs, wet sensations in the genital region, bitter taste in the mouth	Long-Dan-Xie-Gan-Tang

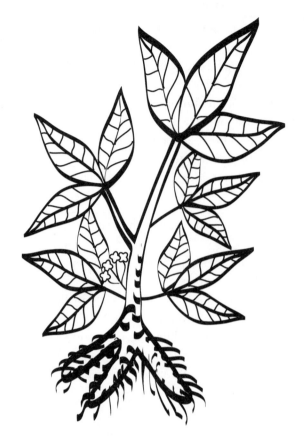

Huang-lian (rhizoma coptidis) **The key ingredient in Huang-Lian-Jie-Du-Tang, an herbal formula effective in treating inflammation and pyogenic infections.**

DISEASE	SYMPTOMS AND SIGNS	HERBAL FORMULAS
Insomnia	falling asleep with difficulty, many dreams and easily disturbed at night, love of sighing, prone to anger, reddish tongue	Dan-Zhi-Xiao-Yao-San
	unable to sleep, mental depression, heaviness in the head, nausea, belching, acid swallowing	Wen-Dan-Tang
	unable to sleep, palpitations, forgetfulness, dizziness, ringing in the ears, dry mouth, night sweats, pain in lower back, reddish tongue	Huang-Lian-E-Jiao-Tang
	many dreams and waking easily, with palpitations, dizziness, fatigue, poor appetite, pale complexion	Gui-Pi-Tang
	sleeplessness with palpitations, nervousness, many dreams, shortness of breath and fatigue	An-Shen-Ding-Zhi-Wan

DISEASE	SYMPTOMS AND SIGNS	HERBAL FORMULAS
Loss of voice	sudden, with cough, nasal congestion, chills or fever	Xing-Su-San
	with sore throat or cough with phlegm	Qing-Yan-Ning-Fei-Tang
	sudden, worsening with stress, sore throat	Xiao-Jiang-Qi-Tang
	hoarseness, with dry throat, sore throat or cough	Sang-Xing-Tang
	chronic, with dry cough and hot palms	Bai-He-Gu-Jin-Tang
Lumbago	pain in the lower back, unable to turn around, worsens on rainy days	Gan-Mai-Ling-Zhu-Tang
	hot pain in the lower back, worse in hot summer, better after moving around	Si-Miao-San
	pricking and fixed pain in the lower back, better during the day and worse at night, with a history of traumatic injury	Shen-Tong-Zhu-Yu-Tang
	mild pain in lower back, relieved by massage and pressure, improves on lying down, recurrent pain	You-Gui-Wan
Nosebleed	with dry nose, dry throat, fever, coughing up scanty phlegm, red tongue	Sang-Ju-Yin
	with bleeding gums, dry nose, bad breath, thirst with craving for drink, constipation, reddish tongue	Yu-Nu-Jian
	with headache and vertigo, prone to anger, pink eyes, bitter taste in the mouth, reddish tongue	Long-Dan-Xie-Gan-Tang
	with bleeding gums, bleeding from muscles, dizziness, ringing in the ears, palpitations, little sleep, pale tongue	Gui-Pi-Tang
Night sweats	sleeplessness, feeling hot, underweight, red cheeks, irregular menstruation in women, seminal emission with erotic dreams in men, reddish tongue	Dang-Gui-Liu-Huang-Tang
	palpitations, little sleep, pale complexion, shortness of breath, fatigue, pale tongue	Gui-Pi-Tang

DISEASE	SYMPTOMS AND SIGNS	HERBAL FORMULAS
Palpitations and nervousness	easily frightened, feeling insecure, many dreams and waking easily	Ping-Bu-Zhen-Xin-Dan
	with dizziness and fatigue, poor complexion	Gui-Pi-Tang
	with ringing in the ears, pain in lower back, hot palms, night sweats	Tian-Wang-Bu-Xin-Dan
	with edema in the lower limbs, nausea and vomiting, chills and cold limbs	Ling-Gui-Zhu-Gan-Tang
	with occasional heart pain, chills and cold limbs, chest discomfort	Tao-Ren-Hong-Hua-Jian
Paralysis	sudden onset in both legs, paralysis of the lumbar spine, thirst, cough, dry throat, reddish urine	Qing-Zao-Jiu-Fei-Tang
	weakness of limbs or numbness, mild swelling with slight heat on touching, love of cold and dislike of heat, mostly affecting the lower limbs	Jia-Wei-Er-Miao-San
	weakened limbs gradually getting worse day by day, poor appetite, watery stools, fatigue, puffy complexion	Shen-Ling-Bai-Zhu-San
	slow onset, affecting the lower limbs, weakened lumbar spine, unable to stand for long or to walk in severe cases, calves deprived of muscles	Hu-Qian-Wan
Perspiration, heavy in the daytime	with aversion to wind, pain all over the body, chills	Gui-Zhi-Tang
	with aversion to wind, particularly when fatigued, susceptible the common cold, fatigue, decreased appetite	Yu-Ping-Feng-San
	as if steaming, fever, reddish complexion, thirst with craving for cold drink, constipation, red tongue	Bai-Hu-Tang
Rheumatism	migratory pain in the joints, stiff joints, chills or fever	Fang-Feng-Tang
	severe and fixed pain in the joints, which may be relieved by heat but intensified by cold	Wu-Tou-Tang
	pain in the joints with swelling, numbness of the skin	Yi-Yi-Ren-Tang
	severe pain in the joints with hot sensations and red swelling in the local region, which may be relieved by cold, fever, aversion to wind, thirst	Bai-Hu-Jia-Gui-Zhi-Tang

DISEASE	SYMPTOMS AND SIGNS	HERBAL FORMULAS
Seminal emission	ejaculation during dreams at night, dizziness, fatigue, reddish tongue frequent ejaculation, bitter taste in the mouth, dry and sticky mouth or ulcer on the tongue, reddish urine, urination problems frequent ejaculation, poor spirits, pale complexion, chills, cold limbs, pain in lower back	Huang-Lian-Qing-Xin-Yin Cheng-Shi-Bie-Xie-Fen-Qing-Yin Bi-Jing-Wan
Skin itch	itch in cold weather (late autumn and winter), dry skin, skin peeling itchy skin in the elderly that gets worse in spring and winter, dry, rough skin, scars caused by scratching, pale tongue itchy skin in young persons, particular in summer and autumn, eczema-like symptoms	Ma-Huang-Tang Si-Wu-Tang Xiao-Feng-San
Stomachache	sudden onset with chills belching or vomiting of undigested foods worsening with stress or anger burning sensation, dry or bitter taste in the mouth in a fixed spot, worsens after eating with dry mouth and craving for drink, constipation	Liang-Fu-Wan Bao-He-Wan Chi-Hu-Shu-Gan-Tang Hua-Gan-Jian Shi-Xiao-San Yi-Wei-Tang
Urinary disorders	scanty urine, hot sensations on urination, abdominal swelling, thirst but no craving for drink, reddish tongue dribbling of urine, shortness of breath, cough, dry throat, thirst with craving for drink diminished urination, mental depression, prone to anger, abdominal swelling, reddish tongue constant desire to pass urine but unable to do so, falling sensation in the lower abdomen, fatigue, poor appetite lack of power to pass urine, lower back pain chills and cold limbs, pale complexion constant desire to pass urine but unable to do so, hot sensations in palms of hand, night sweats, reddish tongue	Ba-Zheng-San Qing-Fei-Yin Chen-Xiang-San Bu-Zhong-Yi-Qi-Tang Shen-Qi-Wan Liu-Wei-Di-Huang-Wan

DISEASE	SYMPTOMS AND SIGNS	HERBAL FORMULAS
Urination, frequent at night	frequent desire to pass urine but unable to finish, hot sensations on urination, mild pain in the lower abdomen	Er-Ding-Tang
	frequent urination at night in large quantity, clear stream of urine, cold limbs, cold lower back pain, fatigue	You-Gui-Wan
	fatigued lower limbs, pale complexion, puffy face and swollen legs, twitching, pale tongue	Da-Ban-Xia-Tang
Vertigo	with ringing in the ears, head swelling, worsens with fatigue or anger, prone to anger, reddish tongue	Tian-Ma-Gou-Teng-Yin
	worsens with movement, often triggered by fatigue, pale complexion, palpitations, poor sleep, pale tongue	Gui-Pi-Tang
	with ringing in the ears, forgetfulness, little sleep, pain in lower back, seminal emission	Zuo-Gui-Wan
	with heavy sensations in the head, chest discomfort, nausea, poor appetite, sleepiness	Ban-Xia-Bai-Zhu-Tian-Ma-Tang

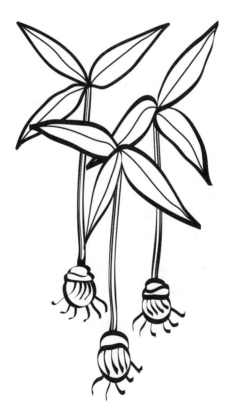

Ban-xia (rhizoma pinelliae)
The key ingredient in Ban-Xia-Hou-Pu-Tang, an herbal formula effective in treating gastrospasm and spasms of the esophagus, nervous exhaustion, and vomiting.

DISEASE	SYMPTOMS AND SIGNS	HERBAL FORMULAS
Vomiting	sudden onset with chest discomfort, chills or fever	Huo-Xiang-Zheng-Qi-San
	with belching that worsens after eating	Bao-He-Wan
	vomiting of clear water or watery phlegm with palpitations or dizziness	Xiao-Ban-Xia-Tang
	with sour taste and belching, chest pain or discomfort	Ban-Xia-Hou-Pu-Tang
	triggered by improper eating, with fatigue and dry mouth	Li-Zhong-Tang
	recurrent, dry vomiting, feeling hungry but no real appetite	Mai-Men-Dong-Tang
Vomiting blood	coughing up blood with food residue in it, bad breath, constipation, reddish tongue	Xie-Xin-Tang
	vomiting of blood in large quantity, bitter taste in the mouth, prone to anger, little sleep with many dreams, reddish tongue	Long-Dan-Xie-Gan-Tang
	chronic vomiting of blood, poor appetite, indigestion, fatigue, palpitations, shortness of breath, pale complexion	Gui-Pi-Tang

CHAPTER 4

Syndromes and Physical Constitution

*A good physician will treat the disease that has not yet occurred,
instead of treating the disease that has already occurred.*
—NEI JING

Symptoms can be classified into thirteen syndromes. By diagnosing the syndrome, a traditional Chinese doctor can prescribe the correct food and herbal cures. For example, anxiety belongs to the nervous syndrome, which should be treated by foods and herbs that calm the spirit, such as apples, cinnamon, and rice and the herbal formulas Suan-Zao-Ren and Zhu-Sha-An-Shen-Wan. The thirteen general syndromes that were established many centuries ago are outlined below, with their symptoms and cures.

COLD SYNDROME

SYMPTOMS	HERBAL CURES	
	HERBS TO USE	**FORMULAS TO USE**
Subjective cold sensations as the key symptom, such as dislike of cold, cold arms and legs, and feeling cold throughout the body	Ma-huang (herba ephedrae), Gui-zhi (ramulus cinnamomi), Cong-bai (allium fistulosum), Gan-jiang (rhizoma zingiberis), Ding-xiang (flos caryophylli)	Apply pungent formulas to warm the body, such as Si-Ni-Tang, Xino-Qing-Long-Tang, and Gui-Fu-Ba-Wei-Wan

Food Cures
Eat warm foods such as caraway seed, chicken, chili pepper leaf and rhizome, chive (Chinese), clove, date, dill seeds, fennel seed, fenugreek seed (Oriental), fresh ginger, green onion (white part), mustard seed, nutmeg, black pepper, white pepper, rice (polished long grain), shallot, sheep or goat's meat and milk, sorghum, star anise, and water chestnut.

HOT SYNDROME

SYMPTOMS	HERBAL CURES	
	HERBS TO USE	FORMULAS TO USE
Subjective hot sensations as the key symptom, such as summer heat, canker sores, sore throat with swelling in the throat, discharge of short streams of red urine	Zhi-mu (rhizoma anemar-rhenae), Shi-gao (gypsum fibrosum), Mu-dan-pi (cortex moutan radicis), Xia-ku-cao (spica prunellae)	Cool the symptoms with cold or cool formulas and formulas to water yin and bring down fire, such as Bai-Hu-Tang, Liu-Yi-Wan, Yin-Qiao-San, and Da-Bu-Yin-Wan

Food Cures

Eat foods with cool or cold energy such as azuki beans, aloe vera, asparagus, bamboo shoot, banana, bitter endive, crab, grapefruit, honey, lemon, mung bean, mung bean sprouts, peppermint, potato, squash, star fruit, sweet basil, and wheat.

LUMPY AND HARD SYNDROME

SYMPTOMS	HERBAL CURES	
	HERBS TO USE	FORMULAS TO USE
Lumpy and hard spots in the body due to energy congestion as the key symptoms, such as hard spots in the abdomen, mass of tissues and swelling in the abdomen with fixed pain. Sometimes, there may be a mass of tissues with wandering pain; also, hard spots in the chest and ribs region, which can be felt only when pain occurs	Cang-zhu (rhizoma atracty-lodis), Hou-pu (cortex magnoliae officinalis), Mu-xiang (radix aucklandiae/radix saus-sureae), Zhi-qiao (fructus aurantii)	Use formulas to soften lumpy and hard spots and attack the affected regions simultaneously, such as Mu-Xiang-Shun-Qi-Wan and Ban-Xia-Tang

Food Cures

Eat foods that have softening properties such as buckwheat, buckwheat sprouts, clam, clam shell powder, crab claws and shell, kelp, kumquat seed, laver, oyster shell, rapeseed (canola), rice bran, and seaweed.

External Attack Syndrome

SYMPTOMS	HERBAL CURES	
	HERBS TO USE	FORMULAS TO USE
When you become sick all of a sudden, it is most likely that you are under the attack of external pathogens, such as the common cold or flu. Most acute diseases fall within this syndrome	Ma-huang (herba ephedrae), Gui-zhi (ramulus cinnamomi), Xi-xin (herba asari), Fang-feng (radix ledebouriellae), Ku-shen (radix sophorae flavescentis)	Use formulas to induce perspiration and transform dampness, such as Ma-Huang-Tang and Xiang-Ru-Yin

Food Cures

Eat antibacterial and antiviral foods such as alfalfa, clove, garlic, ginkgo (fresh), grapefruit, green onion, honeysuckle, hops, jackfruit, kumquat, licorice, mandarin orange, peppermint, purslane, royal jelly, tea, and water chestnuts.

Fatigue Syndrome

SYMPTOMS	HERBAL CURES	
	HERBS TO USE	FORMULAS TO USE
Feeling tired all the time as the key symptom, including dizziness, forgetfulness, weakness of the limbs, a constant desire to rest or lie down	Ren-shen (radix ginseng), Huang-qi (radix astragali seu hedysari), Suan-zao-ren (semen ziziphi spinosae)	Use formulas to warm and rejuvenate, such as Si-Jun-Zi-Tang, Gui-Pi-Tang, and Ren-Shen-Yang-Ying-Tang

Food Cures

Eat foods to boost energy such as beef, cherry, chicken, coconut, date, eel, fermented glutinous rice, ginkgo (cooked), ginkgo root, ginseng, grape, herring, honey, jackfruit, mackerel, mandarin fish, octopus, potato, sweet potato, red and black date, rice (glutinous or sweet rice), shiitake mushroom, squash, string bean root, and white string bean.

CONGESTION SYNDROME

SYMPTOMS	HERBAL CURES	
	HERBS TO USE	**FORMULAS TO USE**
The symptoms refer to lumpy spots due to sputum congestion, as in breast cancer. Sometimes there may be no manifestation of lumpy spots, but you may feel congested	Ting-li-zi (semen lepidii seu descurainiae), Zhu-ru (caulis bambusae in taeniam), Chuan bei mu (bulbus fritillariae cirrhosae), Ban-xia (rhizoma pinelliae), Jie-geng (radix platycodi)	Use formulas to disperse congested symptoms, such as Xiao-Xian-Xiong-Tang and Xiao-Jin-Dan

Food Cures

Eat foods that can eliminate sputum such as almond, apple peel, celery, button mushroom, date, fig, garlic, ginkgo (fresh), grapefruit, honey, jellyfish, kumquat, laver, olive, onion, oyster, peanut, pear, peppermint, radish, rock sugar, sea cucumber, seaweed, shark's fin, shiitake mushroom, sour orange peel, tea, thyme, tofu, walnut, water chestnut, and white sugar.

RETENTION SYNDROME

SYMPTOMS	HERBAL CURES	
	HERBS TO USE	**FORMULAS TO USE**
Retention means to retain something, such as water retention, food indigestion, constipation, suppression of menstruation, etc.	Da-huang (radix et rhizoma rhei), Lu-hui (aloe), Shan-zha (fructus crataegi), Fu-ling (poria), Huo-xiang (herba agastachis), Mu-gua (fructus chaenomelis)	Use formulas to attack and remove water, and induce bowel movements, such as Shi-Zao-Tang, Da-Cheng-Qi-Tang, Zhou-Che-Wan, and Di-Dang-Tang

Food Cures

Eat foods that will eliminate water, promote digestion, and induce bowel movements.

Foods to eliminate water: azuki bean, broad bean, capers, carp (gold), celery, corncob, duck, fenugreek seed (Oriental), fava bean, kelp, mackerel, marjoram, wild oregano, rosin, seaweed, soybean, sweet basil, and watercress.

Foods to promote digestion: buckwheat, carrots, cayenne pepper, coriander, grapefruit, green onion (white part), hawthorn fruit, jackfruit, kiwi fruit, lobster, malt, nutmeg, papaya, peach, quince, radish, sorghum, soybean, sweet basil, tea, tomato, water chestnut, and whitefish.

Foods to induce bowel movements: black sesame seed, cabbage (white), castor bean oil, fenugreek seed (Oriental), fig, papaya, sesame oil, sweet potato, soybean oil, and walnut oil.

DRY SYNDROME

SYMPTOMS	HERBAL CURES	
	HERBS TO USE	**FORMULAS TO USE**
Internal and external dryness as the key symptom, such as thirst, dry skin, and dry constipation	Xuan-shen (radix scrophulariae), Xing-ren (semen armeniacae amarae), Mai-men-dong (radix ophiopogonis), Sha-ren (fructus amomi)	Use formulas to water and moisten internal and external regions of the body, such as Xiong-Yu-Gao, Sha-Shen-Mai-Dong-Yin, and Zeng-Yi-Cheng-Qi-Tang

Food Cures

Eat lubricating foods such as asparagus, banana, cheese, egg (chicken), honey, jellyfish, licorice, milk, peach, pear, peanut oil, pork, sea cucumber, sesame oil, soybean, sugar cane, taro, tofu, and walnut.

SPASTIC SYNDROME

SYMPTOMS	HERBAL CURES	
	HERBS TO USE	**FORMULAS TO USE**
Muscle spasms as the key symptom, including stiffness, lockjaw, stiff neck, twitching of limbs, and tightening of muscles	Tian-ma (rhizoma gastrodiae), Fu-zi (radix aconiti praeparata), Fang-feng (radix ledebouriellae)	Use formulas to relax the spastic symptoms, such as Zi-Shou-Jie-Yu-Tang

Food Cures

Eat foods that induce relaxation such as apple, beer, brown sugar, button mushroom, cantaloupe, cashew, celery, ginseng, hops, jackfruit, longan, nutmeg, rice (polished), rice bran, watermelon, wheat.

Eat antispasmodic foods such as alfalfa, fennel oil, ginkgo leaf, grapefruits, hops, licorice, prickly ash, safflower, shrimp, soybean (black), tomato, wild cabbage.

LOOSE SYNDROME

SYMPTOMS	HERBAL CURES	
	HERBS TO USE	FORMULAS TO USE
Loose refers to symptoms such as excessive perspiration, night sweats, premature ejaculation, chronic diarrhea, and vaginal bleeding	Fu-xiao-mai (fructus tritici levis), Wu-wei-zi (fructus schisandrae), Shan-zhu-yu (fructus corni), Qian-shi (semen euryales), Rou-dou-kou (semen myristicae), Wu-mei (fructus mume)	Use formulas to constrict the symptoms, such as Mu-Li-San, Jin-Suo-Gu-Jing-Wan, and Zhen-Ren-Yang-Zang-Tang

Food Cures

Foods to control urination: bird's nest, cinnamon, ginger (dried), ginkgo (cooked), ginseng, pine mushroom, raspberry, rice (glutinous or sweet rice), strawberry, string bean, tangerine orange peel, walnut, yam.

Foods to stop diarrhea: buckwheat sprout, button mushroom, crabapple, fig, green and dried guava, green prunes, guava (dried), persimmon, pistachio, prunes, quail, rabbit liver, rambutan, rice, sorghum, string bean, sweet potato, and wheat flour.

Foods to control perspiration: rice (glutinous or sweet rice), taro leaf, unripe dried peach, wheat.

DEFICIENT SYNDROME

SYMPTOMS	HERBAL CURES	
	HERBS TO USE	FORMULAS TO USE
Deficient means lacking in energy, including all four kinds of energy: yin energy, yang energy, blood, and vital energy	Ren-shen (radix ginseng), Huang-qi (radix astragali seu hedysari), Shu-di-huang (Radix rehmanniae praeparatae), Bei-sha-shen (radix glehniae), Yin-yang-huo (herba epimedii), Xu-duan (radix dipsaci)	Use formulas to tone the body, such as Liu-Wei-Di-Huang-Wan to tone yin energy, Ba-Zhen-Tang to tone blood and vital energy, Bu-Zhong-Yi-Qi-Tang to tone vital energy, Shen-Qi-Wan to tone yang energy, and Gui-Lu-Er-Xian-Jiao to tone yin energy and yang energy at the same time

Food Cures

Yin tonics: abalone, apple, black-eyed pea, brown sugar, cantaloupe, cheese, clam, coconut milk, crab, cuttlefish, date, duck, egg (chicken and duck), fig, goose, grape, honey, kidney bean, kumquat, lard, lemon, lichee nuts, loquat, mandarin orange, mango, milk, mussel, oyster, pea, pear, pineapple, pomegranate, pork, rabbit, rice (polished), royal jelly, sea cucumber, shrimp, star fruit, string bean, sugar (white), sugar cane, tofu, tomato, watermelon, and yam.

Yang tonics: alfalfa, beef kidney, chicken liver, chive (Chinese), fenugreek seed (Oriental), ginseng, hops, licorice, lobster, mussel, pistachio, pomegranate, raspberry, rosemary, royal jelly, saffron, sardine, sea cucumber, shrimp, soybean, and walnut.

Blood tonics: beef, beef liver, egg (chicken), grape, ham, lichee nuts, longan, milk, octopus, oxtail, oyster, pork liver, sea cucumber, and spinach.

Energy Tonics: beef, cherry, chicken, coconut, date, eel, fermented glutinous rice, ginkgo (cooked), ginseng, grape, herring, honey, jackfruit, longan, mackerel, octopus, pheasant, pigeon (egg and meat), potato, rabbit, rice, rock sugar, shiitake mushroom, squash, sturgeon, sweet potato, and tofu.

PARALYSIS SYNDROME

SYMPTOMS	HERBAL CURES	
	HERBS TO USE	FORMULAS TO USE
Disorders of the motor system as the key symptoms, including paralysis of the four limbs	Xiang-fu (rhizoma cyperi), Chen-pi (pericarpium citri reticulatae), Zhi-shi (fructus aurantii immaturus), Ru-xiang (mastixresina olibaniolibanum), Di-long (lumbricus)	Use formulas to activate energy and blood, such as Xiao-Huo-Luo-Dan and Shu-Feng-Huo-Xue-Tang

Food Cures

Foods to promote blood circulation: brown sugar, cantaloupe, cayenne pepper, celery, chestnut, clam, coriander, crab, eggplant, fermented glutinous rice, green onion, peach, radish, rape (canola), rice (glutinous or sweet rice), saffron, soybean (black and yellow), sturgeon, sweet basil, tofu, turmeric, vinegar, and mustard seed.

Foods to promote energy circulation: beef, black-eyed pea, button mushroom, caraway seed, cardamon seed, carrots, chive (Chinese), clam, dill seeds, egg (chicken), garlic, grapefruit, green onion, hawthorn fruit, jasmine flower, kumquat, lichee, malt, marjoram, mussel, rapeseed, red bean, saffron, shiitake mushroom, spearmint, star anise, string bean, sweet basil, orange peel, tangerine orange and peel, turmeric, and vinegar.

Nervous Syndrome

SYMPTOMS	HERBAL CURES	
	HERBS TO USE	FORMULAS TO USE
Mental disturbances as the key symptoms, including anxiety, nervousness, palpitations, insomnia, many dreams, and convulsion in children	Shi-jue-ming (concha haliotidis), Suan-zao-ren (semen ziziphi spinosae), Bai-zi-ren (semen biotae), Yuan-zhi (radix polygalae), He-huan-pi (cortex albizziae)	Use formulas to sedate and calm the spirits, such as Zhu-Sha-An-Shen-Wan and Bao-Long-Wan

Food Cures

Eat anti-stress and anti-anxiety foods such as apple, bee venom, beer, cantaloupe, cashew, celery, cinnamon, coffee, button mushroom, ginseng, hops, longan, nutmeg, rice (polished), rice bran, watermelon, and wheat.

Treatment of five basic types of physical constitution

It is important to understand your physical constitution—whether you are weak or strong, generally healthy or prone to disease. Foods cannot benefit you unless you know your physical constitution and take it into account when choosing your diet. One serious drawback to the Western theory of nutrition, and modern medicine for that matter, is that it pays almost exclusive attention to the importance of nutritional aspects of foods and ignores the physical constitution of each individual. For example, we are told that it is wise to eat more vegetables because they contain vitamins, or to eat unsaturated fats because they do not increase the cholesterol level, or to cut down on carbohydrates because they contain lots of calories, or to cut down on salt intake because it increases blood pressure. We are told that an ideal diet in the United States contains 10 percent saturated oils, 20 percent unsaturated oils, 12 percent proteins, 40–45 percent complex carbohydrates, and 15 percent sugar. Are those the nutritional goals that all Americans should be aiming to achieve regardless of their physical constitution?

Chinese physicians have classified people into five broad physical constitutions. Each type has its advantages and disadvantages and is predisposed to develop different diseases. The five physical constitutions are: poor circulation type, damp–sputum type, hot–dry type, cold-deficiency type, and fatigue type.

Each constitution is identified through a set of physical traits and symptoms, although some individuals may belong to two or more physical constitutions at the same time. Since each physical constitution is predisposed to develop a number of diseases, different foods are good or bad for different physical constitutions. Therefore, it is important to identify your own physical constitution first, and then identify the foods that are beneficial or detrimental for your type. Identifying your physical constitution and selecting the foods that are good for your type are crucial to using Chinese foods for medicinal purposes.

CLINICAL SIGNS OF PHYSICAL CONSTITUTION

FIVE BASIC TYPES	CLINICAL SIGNS
Dark and obstructive type (energy congestion and blood coagulation)	Dark color of skin, dark color of lips, dark surroundings of the eyes, congested chest, abdominal swelling, deep and retarded and relaxed pulse, blue purple color of the tongue
Water and sputum type (damp sputum type)	Overweight, stomach swelling, sweet taste in the mouth, heavy sensations in the body, discharge of loose stools, thirst with no desire for drink, sliding pulse, greasy coating on the tongue
Dry and hot type or yin deficiency type)	Underweight, dry mouth and dry throat, constipation, internal heat, discharge of short streams of yellowish urine, thirst, insomnia, love of cold drink, ringing in ears, deafness, digestive disorders, wiry and rapid pulse, red color of the tongue with no or little coating on the tongue
Cold and slow type (yang deficiency type)	Overweight, poor complexion, fear of cold, pale lips, cold limbs, excessive perspiration, discharge of loose stools, frequent urination with discharge of long streams of whitish urine, hair loss, ringing in ears, deafness, love of hot drink, deep and weak pulse, light color of tongue with tooth marks on the tongue, tender tongue
Fatigue and deficient type (energy and blood deficiency type)	Pale complexion, shortness of breath, fatigue, dizziness, palpitation, forgetfulness, prolapse of the anus, prolapse of the uterus, excessive perspiration, scanty menstrual flow, numbness of hands, weak and fine pulse, light color of tongue

TREATMENT OF FIVE BASIC TYPES WITH SINGLE HERBS

FIVE BASIC TYPES	HERBS TO USE	HERBS TO AVOID
Dark and obstructive	Chuan-xiong (rhizoma ligustici chuanxiong), Ru-xiang (mastixresina olibaniolibanum), Mo-yao (myrrha), San-leng (rhizoma sparganii), E-zhu (rhizoma zedoariae), Dan-shen (radix salviae miltiorrhizae), Tao-ren (semen persicae), Hong-hua (flos carthami), Pu-huang (pollen typhae), Wu-ling-zhi (faeces trogopterorum)	Di-yu (radix sanguisorbae), Zong-lu-zi (fructus trachycarp)
Water and sputum	Huo-xiang (herba agastachis), Cang-zhu (rhizoma atractylodis), Sha-ren (fructus amomi), Fu-ling (poria), Che-qian (herba plantaginis), Hua-shi (talcum), Mu-tong (caulis aristolochiae manshuriensis), Hou-pu (cortex magnoliae officinalis)	Shu-di-huang (radix rehmanniae praeparatae), Xuan-shen (radix scrophulariae), Mai-men-dong (radix ophiopogonis), Gan-cao (radix glycyrrhizae), Rou-cong-rong (herba cistanchis)
Dry and hot	Bei-sha-shen (radix glehniae), Mai-men-dong (radix ophiopogonis), Tian-dong (radix asparagi), Shu-di-huang (radix rehmanniae praeparatae), Sheng-di (radix rehmanniae), Shi-hu (herba dendrobii), Yu-zhu (rhizoma polygonati odorati), Gui-ban (plastrum testudinis), Bai-he (bulbus lilii)	Gui-zhi (ramulus cinnamomi), Cang-zhu (rhizoma atractylodis), Qiang-huo (rhizoma seu radix notopterygii), Du-huo (radix angelicae pubescentis), Rou-gui (cortex cinnamomi), Ba-ji-tian (radix morindae officinalis)
Cold and slow	Yin-yang-huo (herba epimedii), Tu-si-zi (semen cuscutae), Ba-ji-tian (radix morindae officinalis), Rou-gui (cortex cinnamomi), Fu-zi (radix aconiti praeparata)	Huang-qin (radix scutellariae), Nu-zhen-zi (fructus ligustri lucidi), Bie-jia (carapax trionycis), Ting-li-zi (semen lepidii seu descurainiae), Hua-shi (talcum)
Fatigue and deficient	Shu-di-huang (radix rehmanniae praeparatae), He-shou-wu (radix polygoni multiflori), Bai-shao-yao (radix paeoniae alba), Dang-gui (radix angelicae sinensis), Ren-shen (radix ginseng), Huang-qi (radix astragali seu hedysari), Shan-yao (rhizoma dioscoreae), Da-zao (fructus ziziphi jujubae), E-jiao (colla corii asini/gelatina nigra)	Qiang-huo (rhizoma seu radix notopterygii,), Zhi-shi (fructus aurantii immaturus), Lai-fu-zi (semen raphani), Zi-su-zi (fructus perillae), Quan-xie (scorpio)

TREATMENT OF FIVE BASIC TYPES WITH HERBAL FORMULAS

FIVE BASIC TYPES	HERBAL FORMULAS TO USE
Dark and obstructive	Xue-Fu-Zhu-Yu-Tang, Tong-Qiao-Huo-Xue-Tang, and Yue-Ju-Wan
Water and sputum	Er-Chen-Tang, Ling-Gui-Zhu-Gan-Tang, Wu-Ling-San, and Huo-Xiang-Zheng-Qi-San
Dry and hot	Liu-Wei-Di-Huang-Wan, Yi-Guan-Jian, and Qing-Zao-Jiu-Fei-Tang
Cold and slow	Shen-Qi-Wan, Li-Zhong-Tang, Shen-Fu-Tang, and Bu-Fei-Tang
Fatigue and deficient	Ren-Shen-Yang-Ying-Wan, Sheng-Yu-Tang, Dang-Gui-Bu-Xue-Tang, Bu-Zhong-Yi-Qi-Tang, and Gui-Pi-Tang

FOOD CURES FOR FIVE BASIC TYPES

FIVE BASIC TYPES	FOODS TO EAT	FOODS TO AVOID
Dark and obstructive	See foods under Paralysis Syndrome.	Yin tonic foods (see Deficient Syndrome).
Water and sputum	See foods under Congestion Syndrome and foods under Retention Syndrome.	Greasy foods and yin tonic foods (see Deficient Syndrome).
Dry and hot	See foods under Dry Syndrome and also foods under Hot Syndrome.	See foods under Cold syndrome and Retention Syndrome.
Cold and slow	See foods under Cold Syndrome.	See foods under Hot Syndrome.
Fatigue and deficient	See foods under Deficient Syndrome.	See foods under Congestion Syndrome.

CHAPTER 5

The Healing Effects of Exercise

*Body energy should circulate as regularly and as constantly as the
moon and the sun are circulating without a stop.* —DAO SHU

It's important to your health to lead an active life. The ancient Chinese
put great emphasis on the importance of exercising the body for
longevity. A sixteenth-century Chinese physician named Li Ting said,
"Everyone knows that prolonged walking and standing can cause
excessive fatigue, which is harmful to good health, but few people
mention the harmful effects of lying down or sitting all day." The
Chinese use the term "people of fatigued mind" for people whose days
are spent using their minds—consuming their brain power—and "people of fatigued body" are those who are constantly consuming their
physical energy. The people of fatigued mind, such as scholars, scientists, authors, and white-collar workers, should take steps to tire their
bodies in order to strike a balance between mind and body. The people
of fatigued body, such as farmers, laborers, and blue-collar workers,
should take steps to tire their minds in order to strike a balance
between mind and body. The exercises in this chapter are good for
both types of people, but the people of fatigued mind should do more
of such exercises and more frequently.

Walking

Walking is the simplest form of exercise in traditional Chinese medicine.
It is suitable for all longevity seekers and is a must for older people.
Jogging is not a recommended exercise in traditional Chinese medicine,
but walking, which the Chinese call "relaxed steps," is considered very
important for good health. Unlike jogging, which is intended to tire the
body, walking is intended to relax both the body and the mind.

The Chinese people have always been fond of walking as a means of
promoting good health and longevity. A Chinese political leader in the
modern era was said to be in the habit of walking one mile a day when he

was over 80 years old; another Chinese leader who lived to over 95 walked five hundred steps every day until his death.

How is walking conducive to human health and longevity? The Chinese believe that walking can regulate energy and blood circulation as well as free the mind and body from fatigue. Walking involves bones, muscles, tendons, and blood vessels throughout the body; walking also provides healthy stimulation of internal organs and the brain and regulates the metabolism.

First, walking provides an indirect massage of the internal organs. While you are taking a walk, muscular contraction occurs more often and blood circulation speeds up, in effect massaging the heart indirectly and preventing a decline in the heart's energy. No wonder some scientists believe that walking is the best "heart tonic." Walking can also improve the function of the respiratory system, because physical activities require a greater amount of oxygen to perform. The action of the lungs is believed to double when you're walking compared to when you remain inactive.

Second, walking regulates the metabolism. It has been found that the metabolic rate will increase 75 to 85 percent while a person is walking at a speed of about 50 yards or 160 feet per hour, and it increases by *nine times* when the walking speed doubles. Some metabolic diseases such as diabetes can be prevented simply by walking on a daily basis. For example, in his book published in AD 610, a Chinese physician named Cao Yuan-fang wrote, "A diabetic should walk 120 steps or as many as over 1,000 steps before mealtime." Another Chinese physician, Wang Shou (670–755), said, "It is a good idea to take a walk after meals, rest for a while, and then sit down or lie down."

One study found that after diabetics had traveled for one day on foot, their blood sugar was reduced by 60 mg per 100 mL of blood; by walking two to three miles (four to five kilometers) a day, a person can burn up 300 calories, making walking a good weight-loss exercise. Some Chinese physicians believe that taking a daily walk is the best medicine for regulating metabolism.

Third, walking contains a secret formula for yin tonic. When you feel uneasy, nervous, or tense, your body is shifting toward the yang side, and walking can bring it back to the yin side and strike a balance between yin and yang. Modern medicine would agree, but expresses the concept somewhat differently: walking can reduce muscular tension and relax the nervous system to calm you down. Small wonder that some doctors say walking is the best medicine for nervousness and tension. One doctor reported his experience with patients: When ten of his patients who were too nervous and tense to sleep at night were given sleeping pills, they normally fell asleep within half an hour, but when the patients were instructed to do some light exercises such as taking a walk before bedtime, they fell asleep almost as soon as they went to bed—and the effect lasts longer than sleeping pills.

Fourth, walking is a source of inspiration. Walking improves blood circulation, which is good for inspiration, because when blood circulation is just right, you can think more clearly and effectively. Charles Dickens once said,

> *The sum of the whole is this: walk and be happy; walk and be healthy. The best way to lengthen our days is to walk steadily and with a purpose. The wandering man knows of certain ancients, far gone in years, who have staved off infirmities and dissolution by earnest walking—hale fellows, close upon ninety, but brisk as boys.*

When you are faced with a difficult problem and are anxious to find a solution, take a walk, even inside the office. This often proves effective, perhaps because while you're walking, your cerebral cortex is relaxed temporarily so that it has more room for additional thought. Many scientists and novelists have confessed to having had their best ideas while they were taking walks. Albert Einstein said that every time he came to a blank wall, he took a walk in order to figure out the solution.

As for any exercise intended for health and longevity, you must follow certain rules in order to make the exercise of walking effective. The following are general rules for different types of walking.

The first type of walking, basic walking for good health and longevity, calls for walking 60 to 90 steps per minute for 30 to 60 minutes each day.

The second type of walking, considered good for chronic diseases of the respiratory system, involves walking with both arms swinging back and forth forcefully to engage the shoulders and the chest.

The third type of walking, used widely in traditional Chinese medicine to cure indigestion and other chronic diseases of the digestive system, calls for massaging the abdomen while walking. A Chinese medical classic suggested massaging "the abdomen with both hands while walking over 100 steps to cure indigestion." Once again, modern medicine agrees, proposing that this type of walking can promote the secretion of gastric juices and help empty the stomach, which is a good remedy for indigestion.

The fourth type of walking was originally developed at a health club in Kyoto, Japan, for middle-aged and older people suffering from obesity, hypertension, and other cardiovascular diseases. In this type of walking, over a three-month course of exercise, you must burn up 300 to 500 calories each time you exercise. The intensity of walking is guided by your pulse rate. While walking, people over age 30 should have a pulse rate of 130 beats per minute, people over 40 should have a pulse rate of 120 beats, and those over 60 should have a pulse rate of 110 beats. Each time, the walk should last 30 to 60 minutes on average, to be adjusted up or down according to individual needs. This type of walking is reported to be particularly effective in reducing fat on the abdominal wall and reducing blood pressure.

THE WALKING STYLES OF FIVE ANIMALS

The Chinese exercises popularly known as "the walking styles of five animals" date back to the second century BC, when a Chinese physician named Hua Duo imitated the walking styles of a tiger, a deer, a bear, an ape, and a bird, and recommended them to those who were interested in attaining longevity. He said, "When it comes to exercises for longevity, the walking styles of five animals are very useful, because they are natural ways for the body to move, particularly the waist and the joints, which is an effective way to slow the aging process." The walking styles of five animals have been developed and improved over the centuries.

The walking style of a tiger

STEP 1: With mouth closed, head down, and hands clenched in fists, stand as if you're a tiger about to attack. Lifting your hands very slowly, as if holding something precious, hold your breath, maintain balance in the body, and inhale deeply down to the abdomen, in and out, seven times or until you can hear rumbling in your abdomen.

STEP 2: Again, lift your hands very slowly as if holding something precious, hold your breath, maintain balance in the body, and inhale deeply down to the abdomen, in and out, seven times or until you can hear rumbling in your abdomen.

STEP 3: Move your left foot one step forward, hold out your hands with palms facing to the front, and stand as if you're a tiger about to attack.

STEP 4: Repeat step 2.

STEP 5: Move your right foot one step forward, hold out your hands with palms facing to the front, and stand as if you're a tiger about to attack.

NOTE: This exercise strengthens your hands and feet.

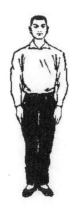 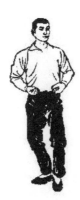 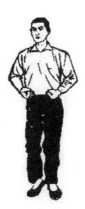 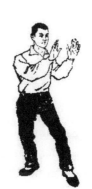 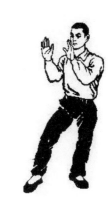

The walking style of a bear

STEP 1: Stand straight, hands hanging naturally at your sides, legs apart. Look straight ahead, inhale deeply three times, and relax.

STEP 2: In a swaying motion, swing the left shoulder toward the left, and slightly bend the left knee.

STEP 3: In a swaying motion, swing the right shoulder toward the right, and slightly bend the right knee.

NOTE: In doing the walking style of a bear, your feet remain on the same spot at all times, and your movements involve all other parts of your body—the waist, shoulder, and legs in particular. Repeat three to five times. This is considered good for strengthening the waist and the tendons.

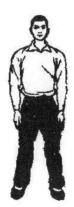 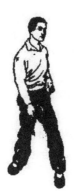 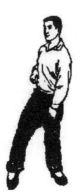

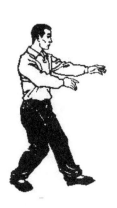

The walking style of a deer

STEP 1: With mouth closed, look straight ahead.

STEP 2: Move the left leg one step forward with the right knee bent and both hands extended forward, palms open.

STEP 3: Jump on tiptoe like a deer.

NOTES: Repeat, alternating the legs. Jumping on tiptoe stengthens the legs.

The walking style of an ape

STEP 1: Stand in the style of the tiger.

STEP 2: Move your left foot one step forward with both knees slightly bent; at the same time, put your left hand forward as if trying to grab something.

STEP 3: Move your right foot one step forward with both knees slightly bent; at the same time, put your right hand forward as if trying to grab something.

Repeat the three steps five times; this style involves the quick movements of hands and feet to strengthen the hands and feet.

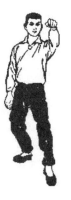
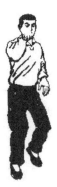

The walking style of a bird

STEP 1: Stand straight, with mouth closed and head up. Look forward and upward as if you were a bird about to fly.

STEP 2: Move your left foot one step forward. At the same time, move your right foot one half step forward, raise your hands, and move your whole body upward as if you were a bird about to fly.

STEP 3: Move you right foot forward so that your two feet are close together, lower your body, with hands crossing each other and upper arms embracing the knees as if you were a bird standing still.

STEP 4: Return to the position in Step 1. Move your right foot one step forward. At the same time, move your left foot one half step forward, raise your hands, and move your whole body upward as if you were a bird about to fly.

NOTE: This style is designed to strengthen the functions of the heart and the lungs; it is also effective in the treatment of lower back pain.

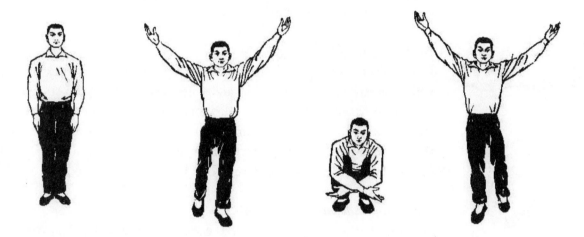

It is important to put yourself in the mind of each animal when doing the exercises above; it is not enough simply to imitate the animal's external movements. In other words, while you're doing these exercises, imagine the psychological state of the animal and focus your inner energy accordingly.

Classic Tai Chi exercises

Tai Chi exercises are more or less a discipline of internal strength. Like the walking styles of five animals, Tai Chi has a long history. This type of exercise is particularly suitable for older people and is considered effective in the prevention of gastrointestinal diseases and hypertension. These exercises can be done with a stick to help you maintain the fixed position of your hands during the exercise; without a stick, you can also imagine that your hands are holding a stick. Three types of Tai Chi exercises use a stick: sitting, reclining, and standing.

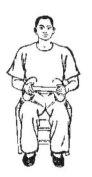

Sitting Tai Chi

Sitting comfortably on a bed or in a chair, hold a 15-inch-long stick between your palms, exerting pressure to hold it steady. Hold the stick a short distance from your navel and push it forward suddenly, which should produce a similar action in the abdomen. The stick should move halfway toward the abdomen without touching it. Repeat 80 to 120 times per minute, and perform 2 to 3 times each day for 2 to 5 minutes each time. After doing the exercise for one to two months, increase the length of time to 5 to 15 minutes each time, and then to 10 to 20 minutes after three months of practice. This type of exercise is particularly good for hiccups, poor appetite, and sleeplessness.

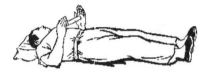

Reclining Tai Chi

Lie comfortably on your back in bed with your head on a thick pillow, your legs stretched out or bent, and your hands holding the stick as in the sitting type of Tai Chi. Rest your arms on your elbows and move the stick back and forth as if rocking a boat (not up and down) 40 to 80 times per minute. Repeat 2 to 4 times, focusing entirely on the navel region. This exercise is considered good for inducing sleep.

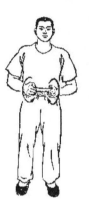

Standing and walking Tai Chi

If you are fairly strong, you can do the standing type of Tai Chi exercises with a stick in the same way as in the lying type or the sitting type. When you do the walking type, turn the stick once each time you walk one step forward, with the knees always slightly bent.

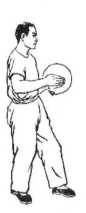
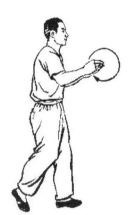

The eight body movements

The eight body movements represent another type of Chinese exercise that dates back 800 years, when they were developed by a group of Chinese physicians in their search for ways to attain longevity. The eight body movements are simpler than the Tai Chi exercises. When practiced forcefully, the eight body movements are more yang than the Tai Chi exercises, but when they are practiced lightly, they are more yin than the Tai Chi movements. The eight body movements are particularly effective in increasing the power of the arms and the muscular strength of the lower limbs, in developing the muscles around the chest, and in preventing curvature of the spine. They are suitable for middle-aged and older persons with chronic diseases.

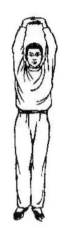

1. Support the heaven with both hands to regulate the "triple heater," or *Sanjiao* (the upper abdomen, middle abdomen, and lower abdomen, all of which produce heat).

   To begin, stand with your arms hanging naturally at your sides, eyes straight ahead. Then do the exercise in the sequences below:
   (a) Lift your arms slowly to the side and continue to lift them until your hands are clasped together over your head, all the while lifting your heels from the ground.
   (b) Turn your palms to face upward, holding your elbows straight and tense. Push your palms upward forcefully, continuing to lift your heels as much as possible. Hold for 30 seconds.
   (c) Relax your fingers and separate your hands. Slowly lower your arms until they are at shoulder height, pointing out, with the heel positions unchanged.
   (d) Lower your heels to the ground and return to the original position.
   Repeat the sequence as many times as you wish, but in general 8 to 16 times are considered adequate; the same holds true for the rest of the eight body movements.

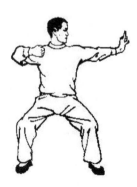

2. Pull the string of a bow toward the left and the right as if about to shoot at a bird of prey.

   To begin, stand straight with the tips of your toes close together. Then do the exercise in the sequence below:
   (a) Move the left foot one step sideways from the center, with both legs bent as if riding a horse, thighs parallel to the ground and the body erect. Cross your arms over your chest, right arm on top

and hands open. Turn your head toward the left, eyes looking at your right hand.

(b) Now clench your left hand into a fist, forefinger up and the thumb straight to form a right angle with the forefinger. Slowly push the left hand outward, extending your left arm straight. At the same time, clench your right hand into a fist and bend the arm, pulling it back horizontally as if you were about to shoot an arrow. The tip of the elbow extends toward the right side and both eyes look straight at the left forefinger.

(c) Open the five fingers of your left fist, pulling the left hand to place it across your chest. At the same time, open the five fingers of the right fist and pull the right hand back to place it across the chest so that the arms cross each other with the left arm on the inside and the right arm on top.

(d) With your right hand in a fist, the forefinger up and the thumb straight to form a right angle with the forefinger, push the right fist outward slowly. Extend the right arm straight, and at the same time, clench the left hand in a fist, with the arm bent and pulling back horizontally as if you were about to shoot an arrow. The tip of the elbow extends toward the left side, and both eyes look straight at the right forefinger.

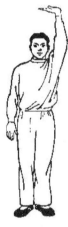

3. Put up one hand to regulate the spleen and stomach.

To begin, stand straight with your arms hanging naturally at your sides. Then do the exercise in the sequence below:

(a) Turn the left palm upward and lift it slowly, with the fingers close together, stretching the left arm as much as possible. At the same time, move the right palm downward and touch the thigh.

(b) Bring your left hand down, with the palm facing downward, to touch the thigh. At the same time, lift your right palm with the fingers close together, stretching the right arm as much as possible with fingertips facing left.

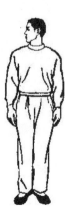

4. Look back to cure five forms of fatigue and seven injuries.

To begin, stand straight with your head upright and arms down, palms touching your thighs. Then do the exercise in the sequence below:

(a) Throw out your chest, with your shoulders bending slightly backward, and turn your head to the left, eyes looking back.

(b) Return your head and shoulders to the original ready position, eyes looking forward.

(c) Throw out your chest, pulling your shoulders slightly toward the back, and turn the head to the right slowly, eyes looking back.

(d) Return your head and shoulders to the original ready position.

5. Shake the head and move the hips ("wag the tail") to clear heart fire.

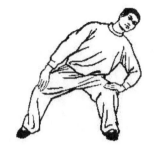

To begin, stand with your legs as wide apart as possible, knees bent as if riding a horse. Hold your knees with both hands, and keeping your upper body straight, do the exercise in the sequence below:

(a) Bend your body as much as possible toward the front left, shaking your head toward the left in a circle and at the same time moving the hips slightly toward the right side in the manner described above, called "wagging the tail"; then return to the original position.

(b) Repeat these movements to the back left, then return to the original position.

(c) Bend your body as much as possible toward the front right, shaking your head toward the right in a circle and at the same time moving your hips slightly toward the left; then return to the original position.

(d) Repeat these movements to the back right, then return to the original position.

6. Touch feet with hands to strengthen the kidney and loins.

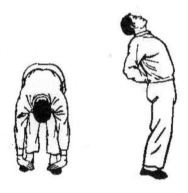

To begin, stand straight and do the exercise in the sequence below:

(a) Bend the upper half of your body forward slowly with knees straight and arms hanging down. Touch your toes or ankles with your hands, lifting your head slightly.

(b) Return to the original ready position.

(c) Place your hands on your back to support the lower back with the palms, and slowly bend the upper half of your body backward.

(d) Return to the original ready position.

7. Clench the fist with an angry look to increase energy.

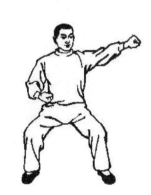

To begin, with legs spread and knees bent as if riding a horse, place your fists on your hips (at the waist), with fists facing upward; then do the exercise in the sequence below:

(a) Slowly but forcefully strike out with your left fist forward and facing down until your arm is straight. With your eyes wide open and looking forward like a tiger, close your right fist tightly, with your elbow pointing backward.

(b) Pull your left fist back to the side of your waist and then return to the original ready position.

(c) Slowly but forcefully strike out with your right fist facing down until your arm is straight. With eyes wide open and looking forward like a tiger, close your left fist tightly, with elbow pointing backward.

(d) Pull your right fist back to your waist and return to the original ready position.

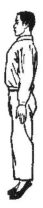

8. Stand on tiptoe and move your head straight upward to cure one hundred diseases.

To begin, stand straight with the tips of your toes close together, hands touching your thighs, and then do the exercise in the sequence below:

(a) Throw out your chest, put your knees close together, and move your head straight upward as if to hit something above. At the same time, lift your heels off the ground.

(b) Lower your heels and return to the original ready position.

Self-massage techniques

Self-massage, a very common practice in many countries, is very useful for relaxation and to alleviate fatigue. The ten massage techniques introduced here are ones you can do by yourself.

Massage your face

(a) Wash your face and comb your hair. Using the center of your palms and starting at your forehead, massage along the sides of your face, downward toward your chin (where the two palms meet). Then from the chin and still using your palms, massage toward the back of your head going up along the ears, brushing through the hair. Return to the forehead to complete the first round of massage. Repeat at least 10 times.

(b) Use the balls of your fingers or fingernails to massage the roots of your hair 10 to 20 times as if combing the hair. Stroke your temple with your thumbs on both sides, gradually moving upward with the other fingers stroking simultaneously, the thumbs and fingers meeting at the top of the head. Next, stroke again toward the back of the head to complete the treatment. This type of self-healing massage is particularly useful to bring down blood pressure, strengthen brain power, cheer yourself up, and reduce wrinkles in the face.

Massage your nose

   (a) With both thumbs slightly bent and the other fingers forming a loose fist, use the backs of the thumbs to rub the nose along the sides from the bridge of the nose to the region below the eyes and downward to the sides of nostrils. Repeat 10 to 30 times.

   (b) Massage the bottom side of the flared portion of each side of the nose with the tip of the thumb and that of the forefinger 10 to 20 times. This is a Chinese acupuncture point traditionally known as "Large Intestine 20" or Li20 for short. Needling this point in acupuncture can cure rhinitis (inflammation of the mucous membrane of the nose). Since this point is particularly effective in increasing the sense of smell or restoring it, the Chinese call this point "greeting scent."

   (c) Massage the philtrum (the groove on the upper lip) with the tip of one finger continually and turning clockwise 50 times and then counterclockwise another 50 times. Then use the ball of the forefinger to press this region 20 times.

An acupuncture point known as D26 in Chinese acupuncture is located slightly above the middle of the philtrum. The Chinese call it "the philtrum point," and as the philtrum looks like a ditch, it is also called "ditch point." Another name for this point is "man in the middle," which refers to a certain passage in the *I Ching*: "There are the way of heaven, way of man, and way of earth." The face of the human body is compared to the universe, which may be divided into heaven and earth, with man in between, so that the forehead is heaven, the chin is earth, and this point is the "man in the middle."

Chinese acupuncturists use this point to cope with emergencies when a patient faints either in the middle of an acupuncture treatment or because of drowning or shock. Some patients are so afraid of acupuncture treatment that they faint when a needle is inserted into the body, so an experienced acupuncturist will insert a needle into this point or simply apply heavy massage to this point with the tip of the forefinger so that the patient wakes up.

When I was in China in October 1985, a 78-year-old Chinese doctor told me that he had made his name as an acupuncturist when he was still a young man just starting his career in a small clinic. On a hot summer day a man suddenly collapsed on the beach because of sunstroke. The man was brought back to the village, but no one was able to wake him up, including a Chinese doctor of Western medicine standing by. A big crowd gathered around the helpless man lying on the ground. This

Chinese acupuncturist happened to be passing by on his way to his clinic, so he took out a needle and inserted it into this acupuncture point. The patient woke immediately.

According to an experiment, when a needle is inserted into this point, it can excite the central nervous system to enhance the respiratory function, cause a rise in blood pressure, and expand the blood vessels in the brain. It has been found to be effective in the treatment of shock and low blood pressure. Lay people can simply massage this point with the tip of the finger to wake themselves up when sleepy or to increase memory power, a very useful technique for students staying up late to study for examinations.

Massage your ears

The Chinese call this massage technique "striking the drum of heaven," because the ears are comparable to a drum and this method involves massaging the ear to make a noise like the striking of a drum. This technique is divided into two steps:

(a) Block both ears with your palms while using three fingers to strike the inion (a point on the external occipital protuberance, the most prominent bone on the back of your head) at least 10 times. Then press the same spot for one minute with the fingers. At the same time, use the palms to block the ears again and then release quickly, which should make noise inside the ears. Do this at least 10 times. Finally, poke the forefingers or middle fingers into the ears and turn the fingers in a circle three times; then remove the fingers and repeat three to five times.

(b) Use the palms to brush the ears until they are hot. Use the forefingers to massage the ear, inside and outside, and pull the ear and its lobe.

Chinese doctors of traditional medicine take human ears very seriously, because they believe that there is an intrinsic connection between the ears and the internal organs. When diseases attack the body, sensitive points will show up in the ears, and by inserting a needle into such sensitive points, the doctors are able to cure such diseases. This is called ear acupuncture in traditional Chinese medicine, now widely used in the West not only to treat diseases but also to help people quit smoking or lose weight. The technique of massaging the ears can increase hearing, improve memory power, and prevent many diseases of the internal organs in general and diseases of the ears in particular.

Rolling and washing the eyes

Traditionally, Chinese doctors believe that many eye diseases can be treated by this method. For example, a Chinese physician in the Ming dynasty (1368–1644) said, "First thing in the morning every day, sit straight and concentrate your thought, rolling both eyes in a circle 14 times. Then close your eyes for a while, and open them quickly. This should cure many eye diseases, including cataracts."

Rolling the eyes: Sit straight and gaze fixedly, with head, back, and waist straight. Look to the left, rolling your eyes in a circle five to six times, then look forward intently for a few seconds. Next, look to the right and roll your eyes in a circle five to six times.

Washing the eyes: Close your eyes and use the balls of your forefingers and middle fingers of both hands to massage the lower edge of your eyeballs in a circle 10 times as if washing the eyes with water, and then repeat in the opposite direction in a circle 10 times. Next, use the ball of the forefinger to massage the inner and outer angles of both eyes and the temple point on both sides. The temple point is important in Chinese acupuncture, effective in the treatment of eye diseases and headaches, particularly migraine headache.

Exercising and washing the eyes can help develop strong eye muscles; improve the functions of the oculomotor nerve, which is distributed through the muscles of the eye; and improve the function of the optic nerve, which consists of sensory fibers that conduct impulses from the eye to the brain. The same technique can also promote blood circulation in the eyeball orbit tissues, which is considered useful in preventing such eye conditions as squint, nearsightedness, and farsightedness.

Qi Gong exercises

Qi means energy, *Gong* means discipline; *Qi Gong* means the discipline of energy. There are three way to discipline your body energy: first, relax your body so that your body energy can be controlled more easily; second, use your will to direct the movements of your body energy; third, direct your body energy to move to a certain region of your body in order to treat the symptoms in that particular region, such as pain in the right ankle or numbness in your fingers.

Qi Gong may be practiced in a number of postures: lying on your side, lying on your back, sitting, or lying on your back with your head on a pillow.

Lying on side

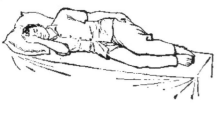

In this posture, your head should bend forward slightly and be supported firmly by a pillow so that it won't move. The spine should bend slightly backward for comfort. If you are lying on your right side, your right hand should be bent a little bit, with all five fingers stretched comfortably and the palm facing upward and placed a short distance from the ear, in front of the ear and on the pillow. The left hand remains open, with all five fingers open and relaxed, palm facing downward, placed on the left hip. The right leg is stretched naturally, with the left knee joint at 120 degrees and placed lightly on top of the right leg (reverse the posture when lying on left side). Both eyes should remain closed or slightly open; the mouth opens and closes as you breathe.

Lying on back

In maintaining this posture, your head should bend forward slightly, the torso remains straight, and your arms are stretched naturally and comfortably. All 10 fingers are relaxed, the palms face downward and are placed at the sides, the lower limbs are stretched naturally, the heels are close together, and the toes of the feet are separated from each other. Both eyes should remain closed or slightly open; the mouth opens and closes in tune with respiration.

Lying on back with head on the pillow

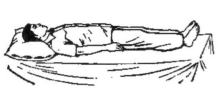

The requirements for lying on your back with your head on the pillow are basically the same as for lying on your back, the only difference being that your head is supported by a pillow so that it is slightly higher than your shoulders, with no empty space under your neck. Palms firmly on the thighs, and the legs are closed together.

Sitting

Sit straight in a chair with your head bent forward slightly, torso straight, shoulders relaxed, hands down, fingers stretched and relaxed comfortably, palms facing downward and placed on your upper legs. The feet are parallel to each other and as far apart as the shoulders. Your lower legs meet the ground at right angles, with knee joints forming a 90-degree angle. If the chair is too high or too low to be able to sit this way, put a cushion on the chair or under your feet. Both eyes should remain closed or slightly open to see only a dim light; the mouth opens and closes in tune with the act of respiration.

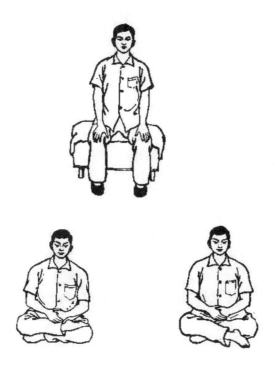

Tips on how to practice Qi Gong

In general, you should start from a lying posture, because the sitting posture may make you tired and cause backache. However, the lying postures will also cause discomfort if they are practiced for an extended period. The important thing to remember is that you should never try to continue in the same posture if you are feeling uncomfortable; change positions to make your body more comfortable.

Which lying posture should be adopted depends on your physical condition and preference. For example, if you have a weak stomach with slow bowel movements and evacuation, lying on your right side would be a good choice, particularly when doing these exercises after meals. The postures in which you lie on your back or side may be used together or singly with similar results, although lying on your back with your head on the pillow, unlike the lying on back posture, should be adopted later as the practice continues, as it is stronger in effect.

After you've practiced the two lying postures for about ten days, you should find that the strength of your body has increased considerably. You can now add the sitting posture to the practice so that two different types of postures are used alternately, with use of the sitting posture gradually increased. As a rule, the sitting posture should be used first each time, to be followed by the lying posture. When practiced after meals, however, the lying posture may be used first, to be followed by the sitting posture. Whatever postures you use, gradually extend the duration each time but not to the point of fatigue.

How to control breathing

Close the mouth and inhale through the nose. Concentrating intently, direct the air to the lower abdomen and hold it there, then exhale slowly. The entire process may be divided into "inhale, stop, exhale." The acts of breathing may be coordinated by quietly saying a different word or words at the beginning of each action, like "inhale," "stop," "exhale"; gradually increase the number of words but don't exceed nine words. The words you choose should have something to do with quietude, relaxation, health, beauty, harmony, and so on. For example, you can use "calming myself," or "I am relaxing," or "exercising to relax," "relaxing my brain," or "I am determined to be healthy," and so on. If your three words were "calming myself down," you would murmur "calming" while you were inhaling, "myself" while you were holding your breath, and "down" while you were exhaling. The movements of the tongue are also important while you are doing this exercise: lift the tongue to touch the front upper gums while inhaling, hold the tongue still while holding the breath, and relax the tongue while you're exhaling.

Inhale through the nose or through the nose and the mouth. Inhale first without stopping and then exhale and stop. The process may be divided into inhale, exhale, stop, accompanied by murmuring words as before. Lift the tongue to touch the front upper gums while inhaling, slowly lower the tongue while exhaling, with the tongue staying still while stopping.

This third exercise is more difficult to master. This time, as described below, you will inhale and then exhale slowly with no stopping in between, but you will stop during the inhalation in a process divided into inhale, stop, continue to inhale, exhale. Try to murmur only three words as described in the following instructions:

Inhale a little bit through the nose and then stop; lift your tongue to touch the front upper gums and murmur the first word while inhaling; stop, hold your tongue, and murmur the second word. Inhale more air in larger quantities and, concentrating intently, direct the air to the lower abdomen, while murmuring the third word.

In general, the first two methods for controlling breathing are used more often than the third. The first may cause a number of symptoms involving the head, chest, and abdomen, because it breaks with the normal type of natural breathing in daily life; for that reason, you should proceed gradually without forcing yourself to practice too much, to let the body adjust to it. The second is very close to the normal type of natural breathing in daily life, and for that reason it can be practiced fairly easily and more often.

Those who suffer from psychological tensions and slower gastrointestinal functions may find it helpful to practice the first method, because when the breathing comes to a stop, the exhaling that immediately follows is enhanced and excites the parasympathetic nerves, which dilate blood vessels, slow the heart rate, and stimulate secretions.

If you become dizzy and experience discomfort in the stomach and intestines after practicing the first method, use the second method. When the breathing comes to a stop after exhaling, the inhaling that immediately follows is enhanced and excites the sympathetic nerves, which cause contraction of blood vessels, increase the heart rate, and inhibit stomach and glandular secretions.

Whichever method of breathing you use, always obey the principle of proceeding naturally and gradually. In addition, the acts of sending air deep down to the lower abdomen, murmuring words, and moving the tongue should be coordinated well, something beginners often fail to achieve. Therefore, it is a good idea to do the exercises step by step. Start from the easiest exercise and work toward the most difficult. First, coordinate the acts of breathing with murmuring the words. Also, murmuring should be done simultaneously in thought and sounds; it is basically designed to bring all distracting thoughts together and transform them into an intent concentration that will provoke corresponding physiological change. Moreover, the words you select should be based on your symptoms and physical condition.

When psychological tensions are present, murmur, "Relax" or "I am relaxing." When indigestion and other digestive disturbances occur, murmur, "Stomach gets going." When anemia and fatigue are present, murmur, "Tranquillity produces true energy," or "Exercises producing energy and blood." When chest congestion and abdominal swelling are present, murmur, "Exercises releasing congestion," and the like. It must be pointed out, however, that the act of murmuring is intended only to increase the ability to concentrate, not to regulate the speed of breathing.

Intent concentration

Intent concentration means to focus attention on something in order to do away with extraneous thoughts. This allows you to focus your attention fully on the exercises. A number of methods for achieving intent concentration are discussed below.

The "field of magic pills"

The field of magic pills is located just below the navel. It coincides with an acupuncture point called "sea of energy" known to Western acupuncturists as R6. When the air, called "the energy of space" in the Chinese language, is sent to the lower abdomen, it gathers at this point and becomes the sea of the energy of space. The sea of energy is related closely to the act of breathing, because air does not reach as far down as the lower abdomen in normal breathing. In practicing the art of Qi Gong, however, this point should be activated so that air can be sent to the lower abdomen. Although an acupuncture point is a very tiny point on the skin, for the purpose of practicing intent concentration on the field of magic pills, you should imagine this spot to be a round, flat surface or a spherical container instead.

The midpoint between nipples or the pit of the stomach

The midpoint between nipples is another acupuncture point, known to Western acupuncturists as R17, and it is an effective point for diseases of the lungs.

The big toe

With both eyes slightly closed, gaze at the big toe and focus your attention on it. Or, with both eyes closed, focus your thoughts on the big toe.

In general, intent concentration on the field of magic pills is relatively stable and will not produce any symptoms in the head, chest or abdomen. However, some women have found that practicing this type of exercise leads them to develop either excessive menstrual flow or prolonged menstruation. In such cases, intent concentration on the midpoint between nipples should be practiced instead. Some people find it extremely difficult to concentrate due to the presence of many distracting thoughts, in which case intent concentration on the big toe should prove easier than the two preceding methods. It should not, however, be practiced all by itself. Rather, two or three methods should be practiced alternately. Like other types of exercises, intent concentration should be practiced in moderation with thoughts neither too concentrated nor too distracted.

Precautions

The exercises introduced so far are useful not only in nourishing internal energy to relieve psychological tension and promote clear thinking, they can also regulate the disturbances of the digestive system. Many practitioners experience a dramatic increase in appetite and digestion. If this occurs, you should increase food intake gradually, particularly if you are underweight; refrain from overeating and from doing exercises on an empty stomach.

Walk around the room for five minutes before starting the exercises. Gargle with a little water and then swallow it all the way to the field of magic pills to help calm you down to get ready for the exercises. If, in the middle of exercises, you feel discomfort in the chest, stop the exercise, walk a few steps, and drink a little water, then start all over again in a few minutes. After each period of exercise, routinely rub the face and abdomen, and rock the body back and forth as closing movements.

Active Tai Chi

Step One: getting started

DIAGRAM 1: Stand straight, feet as wide apart as the shoulders, toes pointing forward, arms at the side, eyes looking straight ahead.

DIAGRAMS 2–3: Slowly extend the arms forward until they are level with the shoulders, palms facing down.

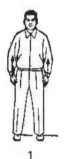 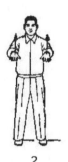 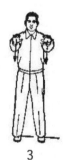

1   2   3

DIAGRAM 4: The body remains straight, with knees bent and palms pressing downward, elbows down and knees aligned, eyes looking straight ahead.

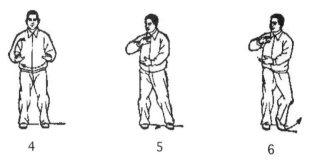

Step Two: wild horse separating mane

DIAGRAMS 5–6: The upper body turns slightly to the right, with the center of gravity shifting to the right thigh, at the same time bring the right arm to the front of the chest, palm facing downward, moving the left hand in front of the chest to stop below the right hand by moving in the form of an arc, the palm of hand facing upward, two palms facing each other as if holding a ball; bring the left foot to the medial side of the right foot, standing on tiptoe, eyes looking at the right hand.

DIAGRAMS 7–9: The upper body turns slightly to the left, the left foot steps forward toward the left, with the center of gravity on the heel of the right foot, extending the right leg naturally, the left leg forming an arc; at the same time, the upper body continues to turn left, the hands separate from left upward and toward the right downward, the left hand remains on a level with the eyes (palm of hand angled upward), elbow slightly bent, the right hand lands on the right hip, the elbow slightly bent, palm of hand facing downward, fingertips forward, eyes looking at the left hand.

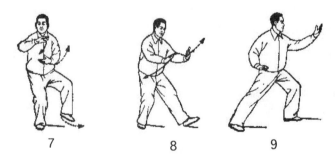

DIAGRAMS 10–12: The upper body slowly moves backward with the center of gravity shifting to the right leg, tip of left foot up and slightly angled (about 45 to 60 degrees); the left foot slowly lowers, the body turning left, the center of gravity shifting to the left leg again, and in the meantime the left hand moving to face downward, putting the left arm in front of the chest; the right hand moving toward the left to place below the left hand with two hands forming an arc, palms facing each other as if holding a ball; place the right foot on the medial side of the left foot, standing on tiptoe with eyes looking at the left hand.

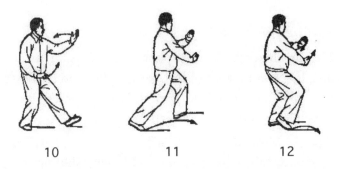

10   11   12

DIAGRAMS 13–14: Move the right leg forward, then extend the left leg naturally to form an arc, and in the meantime turn the upper body toward the right, hands slowly moving down to the left and up to the right respectively, with the right hand on a level with the eyes (palm of hand angled upward), elbow slightly bent, left hand lands on the left hip, elbow slightly bent, palm facing down, fingertips forward, eyes looking at the right hand.

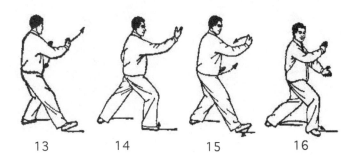

13   14   15   16

DIAGRAMS 15–17: the same as Diagrams 10–12 except in the opposite direction.

DIAGRAMS 18–19: the same as Diagrams 13–14 except in the opposite direction.

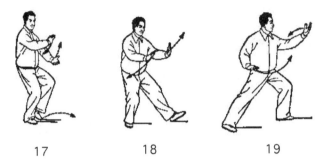

17   18   19

Step Three: white crane shining her wings

DIAGRAM 20: The upper body turns left, the left palm turns to face downward, left arm in front of the chest, right hand moves to upper left to draw an arc, palm of hand turn to face upward, as if two hands holding a ball, eyes looking at the left hand.

DIAGRAMS 21–22: Move the right foot half a step forward, move the upper body backward with the center of gravity shifting to the right leg, upper body turns right, with the face in the right-front direction, eyes looking at the right hand, left foot moves slightly forward, toes touching the ground very lightly, and in the meantime, turn the upper body to the left, facing the front, moving two hands separately in the upper right and lower left directions, and move the right hand upward to stop in front of the right side of forehead, palm of hand facing the left back, the left hand lands in front of the left hip, palm facing downward, fingertips facing front, eyes looking forward.

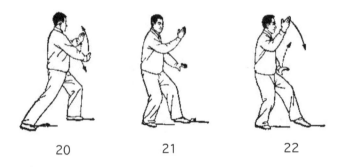

20   21   22

CHAPTER 6

Treatment of Common Diseases in Western Medicine

The real misery of a human being is being vulnerable to all kinds of diseases; the real misery of a doctor is lacking in effective treatments of diseases. —SHI JI

The digestive system

ALLERGIC ENTERITIS

Allergic enteritis is a nonspecific inflammatory disease that affects the small intestine and causes diarrhea. In traditional Chinese medicine, it is believed that this disease affects the liver and spleen in particular. There are two distinct syndromes of this disease.

SIGNS AND SYMPTOMS	SYNDROMES AND TREATMENT
Chest discomfort and poor appetite, diarrhea, edema, jaundice, nausea, or vomiting	Spleen dampness syndrome: Si-Jun-Zi-Tang or Shi-Pi-Yin
Chronic backache, deafness, diarrhea, toothache, hair loss, white vaginal discharge, frequent miscarriage or inability to conceive in women	For kidney efficiency: Bu-Shen-Tang

CIRRHOSIS

Cirrhosis is a disease of the liver that results in chronic damage to the liver cells, with bands of fibrosis breaking up the normal structure of the liver. Common causes of cirrhosis are heavy alcohol consumption and hepatitis, particularly hepatitis B. There may be no symptoms, but the common symptoms are mild jaundice, edema, mental confusion, vomiting of blood, and enlargement of the liver and spleen on examination. The diagnosis is usually confirmed by a liver biopsy. In traditional Chinese medicine, it is believed that this disease affects the liver, the spleen, and the kidneys in particular. There are six syndromes to be considered.

SIGNS AND SYMPTOMS	SYNDROMES AND TREATMENT
Thick greasy coating on the tongue, abdominal pain with rumbling, blisters on the skin, chest discomfort, diarrhea, diminished urination, dizziness, eczema, swollen feet, a heavy sensation in the body, watery stools, illness starting mostly from the lower regions of the body, toes extraordinarily itchy	Dampness syndrome: Wei-Ling-Tang
Glossy and moist coating or white coating on the tongue, abdominal pain, chest pain, constipation, stomachache, swallowing difficulty, swelling and congestion after eating, breast swelling in women	Energy congestion: Wei-Ling-Tang
Abdominal pain, abnormal perspiration, diarrhea, low-grade fever, burning sensation and itch in the genitals, jaundice, red and painful eyes, watering eyes, intolerant to light, cracked lips, red and scanty urine, swollen tongue, thick and sticky vaginal discharge with an offensive odor	Superficial damp-heat or damp-heat flowing downward syndrome: Si-Jun-Zi-Tang with Si-Ling-San or Shi-Pi-Yin
Thick and greasy coating on the tongue, diarrhea, edema, jaundice, nausea and vomiting, sweet-sticky taste in the mouth, fatigue, plentiful vaginal discharge in women	Spleen dampness: Si-Jun-Zi-Tang with Ping-Wei-San

CIRRHOSIS (continued)

SIGNS AND SYMPTOMS	SYNDROMES AND TREATMENT
Thin layer of white coating or white-greasy coating on the tongue, light color of the tongue, fat and tender tongue with tooth marks along edge, shivering with cold sensations of limbs, lower back pain, diarrhea at dawn or chronic diarrhea, scanty urine with puffiness, pale complexion	Yang deficiency of the spleen and the kidneys: Fu-Zi-Li-Zhong-Tang with Si-Ling-San
Red tongue with scanty coating of the tongue, dizziness, ringing in ears, hot sensations in the palms of hands and the soles of feet or numbness of limbs, difficulty in flexing and extending, jumping of muscles, seminal emission in men, scanty menstrual flow and suppression of menstruation in women	Deficiency of the liver and the kidneys: Liu-Wei-Di-Huang-Wan with Si-Ling-San

GALLSTONES

Gallstones are round or oval pieces of solid matter in the gallbladder. They may also be found in the bile ducts, where they cause severe symptoms. Gallstones are composed primarily of cholesterol, but some may contain a large amount of bile pigments and other substances, such as calcium compounds. Only about 20 percent of gallstones cause symptoms, which develop when a gallstone gets stuck in the bile duct. This may cause biliary colic, which involves intense pain in the upper right side of the abdomen or between the shoulder blades. About 95 percent of gallstones may be detected by ultrasound scanning. Gallstones may be left alone when they do not cause symptoms.

SIGNS AND SYMPTOMS	SYNDROMES AND TREATMENT
Bitter taste in the mouth, deafness, pain in the ribs	Heat attacking gallbladder meridian: Da-Chai-Hu-Tang

GALLSTONES (continued)

SIGNS AND SYMPTOMS	SYNDROMES AND TREATMENT
White coating on the tongue, pain in lower abdomen affecting the testes in men, falling of the scrotum with hardness and swelling and pain, cold limbs	Cold accumulation in the liver meridian: Wu-Zhu-Yu-Tang or Chai-Hu-Gui-Jiang-Tang

CHRONIC GASTRITIS

Chronic gastritis is chronic inflammation of the mucous membrane that lines the stomach; it develops gradually over a long period. The common symptoms include discomfort in the upper abdomen, nausea, and vomiting, which are often aggravated by eating. Common causes of chronic gastritis include prolonged alcohol and tobacco use, which causes irritation and aging.

SIGNS AND SYMPTOMS	SYNDROMES AND TREATMENT
Thick and greasy coating on the tongue, diarrhea, edema, jaundice, nausea and vomiting, sweet-sticky taste in the mouth, fatigue, plentiful vaginal discharge in women	Spleen dampness syndrome: Si-Jun-Zi-Tang with Ping-Wei-San to strengthen the spleen and dry the dampness
Light color of the tongue with white and greasy coating, abdominal pain, love of heat and warmth, hiccups, vomiting, poor appetite, abdominal swelling after a meal, fatigue, weakness, cold limbs or scanty urine and puffiness, whitish vaginal discharge in women	Deficiency coldness of the spleen and the stomach: Xiang-Sha-Liu-Jun-Zi-Tang to strengthen the spleen and harmonize the stomach

ACUTE GASTROENTERITIS

Acute gastroenteritis is an acute inflammation of the stomach and intestines that may give rise to many forms of stomach upsets. Common symptoms are loss of appetite, nausea, vomiting, cramps, and diarrhea; common causes include bacteria, bacterial toxins, viruses, contaminated food and water, and alcohol and drugs.

ACUTE GASTROENTERITIS (continued)

SIGNS AND SYMPTOMS	SYNDROMES AND TREATMENT
Blisters in the middle of the tongue, yellow coating on the tongue, abdominal swelling and obstruction, burning sensation in the anus, diarrhea of deep-yellow stools with an offensive smell, poor appetite, yellowish urine, vomiting of sour decomposed foods and liquids	Spleen-stomach damp heat: Huo-Xiang-Zheng-Qi-San with Liu-Yi-San; or use Can-Shi-Tang to clear heat and dampness
Light color of the tongue with white coating, abdominal pain, love of heat and warmth, hiccups, vomiting of clear water and undigested foods, poor appetite, abdominal swelling after a meal, fatigue, cold limbs or scanty urine and puffiness, whitish vaginal discharge in women	Deficiency coldness of the spleen and the stomach: Si-Ni-Tang, Li-Zhong-Tang, or Ji-Bao-Yu-Gua-Tang; or Huo-Xiang-Zheng-Qi-San to warm the middle region

CHRONIC HEPATITIS

Hepatitis is an inflammation of the liver developed over a long period; it is mostly caused by heavy alcohol consumption or a reaction to a medication. Normally, a vague feeling of illness is the common symptom. On examination, the liver may be found to be enlarged, and a virus or antibody may be found in the blood.

SIGNS AND SYMPTOMS	SYNDROMES AND TREATMENT
Greasy or white coating on the tongue, absence of perspiration in hot weather. Cold sensations in the lower abdomen–genitals region, diarrhea, edema in the four limbs, pain in the body or the joints, scanty and clear urine, stomachache, menstrual pain in women	Cold-dampness syndrome: Yin-Chen-Zhu-Fu-Tang to warm and transform cold and dampness

CHRONIC HEPATITIS (continued)

SIGNS AND SYMPTOMS	SYNDROMES AND TREATMENT
Red tongue with tooth marks visible, constipation, fatigue, dry mouth, mild stomachache with swelling, palpitations, scanty urine, thirst, fever in the afternoon	Simultaneous deficiency of yin and energy: Chai-Hu-Shu-Gan-Tang with Da-Bu-Yin-Wan to treat it
Purple-dark color of the tongue or hemorrhages on the tongue, abdominal swelling, congested chest, lump in the abdomen, pain in the chest with a lumpy sensation and pricking pain	Energy stagnation and blood coagulation (energy congestion may cause blood coagulation and vice versa, which is why the two syndromes often occur simultaneously): Xiao-Yao-San with Tao-Hong-Si-Wu-Tang to disperse the liver, regulate energy, activate blood, transform coagulation
White-greasy coating on the tongue, swelling of rib regions, poor appetite, congested sensations in the stomach, stomachache, belching, acid swallowing, nausea, vomiting, abdominal swelling, intestinal rumbling, watery stools	Disharmony between the liver and the spleen: Si-Jun-Zi-Tang with Jin-Ling-Zi-San to disperse liver and strengthen the spleen
Greasy or white coating on the tongue, light color of the tongue, abdominal pain, diarrhea, edema, hiccups, plenty of saliva, stomachache	Spleen-stomach deficiency syndrome: Xiang-Sha-Liu-Jun-Zi-Tang to strengthen the spleen and harmonize the stomach

The respiratory system

BRONCHIAL ASTHMA

Bronchial asthma is the narrowing of small airways in the lungs, called "bronchioles," with recurrent attacks ranging from mild breathlessness with wheezing, particularly on exhaling, to respiratory failure. Bronchial asthma is divided into two types: one is extrinsic, occurring when an allergy caused by something like pollen, dust, or animals triggers an attack; the other is intrinsic, in which there is no external cause.

SIGNS AND SYMPTOMS	SYNDROMES AND TREATMENT
Light-red color of the tongue, thin white coating on the tongue, absence of perspiration in hot weather, clear discharge from the nose, aversion to cold, headache, stuffed nose	Wind-cold syndrome: Xiao-Qing-Long-Tang to disperse wind and cold, drive out sputum, and calm asthma
Light-white color of the tongue, swollen tongue, abdominal rumbling, headache with dizziness, pain in the chest and the ribs, palpitations	Sputum syndrome: San-Zi-Yang-Qin-Tang with Ting-Li-Da-Zao-Xie-Fei-Tang to drive out sputum, bring down energy, and calm asthma
Red tongue, yellowish and greasy coating on the tongue, cough. Discharge of hard yellow sputum in lumps, cloudy and thin stools with an offensive odor, insomnia, vomiting, wheezing	Hot sputum: Xiao-Qing-Long-Jia-Shi-Gao-Tang
Dry and red tongue, greasy yellow coating on the tongue, pain in the chest, pain in the throat with dry sensations, exhaling hot air from the nose, urgent panting, yellowish urine	Hot lung: Ma-Xing-Gan-Shi-Tang to treat it in case of fever; or Ding-Chuan-Tang to treat it if no fever is observed
Light color of the tongue, white coating on the tongue, fatigue, fear of cold, low and weak voice, perspiring easily, shallow and intermittent breathing without lifting the shoulders, withered and pale complexion	Lung deficiency: Yu-Ping-Feng-San to tone the lungs and solidify the superficial region
Glossy or white coating on the tongue, light color of the tongue, cold abdominal pain or swelling with a fondness for massage, fatigue, indigestion, poor appetite, prolonged diarrhea with muddy stools	Spleen energy deficiency: Liu-Jun-Zi-Tang to strengthen the spleen and benefit energy

BRONCHIAL ASTHMA (continued)

SIGNS AND SYMPTOMS	SYNDROMES AND TREATMENT
Lower back pain, weak legs, dizziness, visual whirling sensations, ringing in the ears, deafness, seminal emission in men, suppression of menstruation in women, infertility, night sweats, dry sensations in the mouth with no desire for drink, red tongue	Yin deficiency of the kidneys: Liu-Wei-Di-Huang-Wan to water yin and tone the kidneys
Panting, shortness of breath, weak loins and knees, fatigue, excessive perspiration, weak voice, greenish complexion, cold limbs, fear of cold, wheezing	Loss of kidneys' capacity: Shen-Qi-Wan to tone the kidneys and increase the capacity

BRONCHIECTASIS

Bronchiectasis is a lung disease in which the bronchi are distorted and stretched. It may cause a cough that produces green or yellow sputum with flecks of blood, accompanied by shortness of breath. It is mostly caused by childhood chest infections and is normally diagnosed from the symptoms.

SIGNS AND SYMPTOMS	SYNDROMES AND TREATMENT
Red tongue, yellowish and greasy coating on the tongue, cough, discharge of hard yellow sputum in lumps, discharge of cloudy and thin stools with an offensive odor, insomnia, vomiting, wheezing	Hot sputum: Wei-Jing-Tang to clear the lungs and transform sputum
Red color of the tongue and slightly coated, coughing out blood, dry sensations in the mouth, hoarseness, night sweats, insomnia, sputum with blood	Lung yin deficiency: Sha-Shen-Mai-Dong-Tang to nourish the lungs

BRONCHIECTASIS (continued)

SIGNS AND SYMPTOMS	SYNDROMES AND TREATMENT
Abundant saliva, overweight but intake of only a small amount of food, slight fullness of the stomach, suppression of menstruation in women, weakened limbs	Spleen sputum: Liu-Jun-Zi-Tang to strengthen the spleen and transform sputum. This type of bronchiectasis is stable with mild symptoms
Red color of the tongue, cough with scanty sputum, dry sensations in the mouth at night, night sweats, seminal emission with dreams in men, underweight, insomnia	Lung kidney deficiency: Sheng-Mai-San or Shen-Ge-San to benefit the kidneys and tone the lungs

ACUTE BRONCHITIS

Acute bronchitis develops quickly and usually clears up within a few days. The primary symptoms are wheezing, shortness of breath and cough with sputum, caused by a viral infection such as a cold or flu, pollutants, or a bacterial infection. In traditional Chinese medicine, it is believed that this disease involves cough due to the attack of external pathogens.

SIGNS AND SYMPTOMS	SYNDROMES AND TREATMENT
Glossy and moist coating of the tongue, light red color of the tongue, absence of perspiration in hot weather, clear discharge from nose, cough, diarrhea, dislike of cold, headache with dizziness, hoarseness, nosebleed, pain in the joints, stuffed nose, vomiting	Wind-cold: Xing-Su-San to disperse wind and cold, expand the lungs, and suppress cough
Cough or coughing out blood, dizziness, headache with dizziness, yellowish discharge from the nose, nosebleed, red and painful eyes, sore throat, thirst, toothache, yellow urine	Wind-heat: Sang-Ju-Yin to disperse wind, clear heat, expand the lungs, and transform sputum

ACUTE BRONCHITIS (continued)

SIGNS AND SYMPTOMS	SYNDROMES AND TREATMENT
Red color of the tongue with yellow coating, constipation, cough, dry lips, dry sensations in the mouth, high fever, profuse perspiration, scanty urine, thirst	Summer heat: Xiang-Ru-Yin with Jie-Geng-Tang to disperse wind, clear the lungs, and relieve summer heat
Swollen tongue with a black coating, abdominal pain, absence of perspiration in hot weather, absence of thirst, abundant watering of eyes, clear and long urine in large quantities, whitish urine	External cold: Zhi-Sou-San to stop cough, expel cold, and transform phlegm
Inability to extend the tongue, cold hands and feet, cold fingertips, hot sensations in the center of palms and the soles of feet	Internal heat: Ma-Xing-Gan-Shi-Tang to induce perspiration and clear the lungs
Red color of the tongue with a thin layer of yellow coating, constipation, cough, fatigue, high fever, obstructed urination with red urine, profuse perspiration, poor appetite, thirst	Summer heat: Xiang-Ru-Yin with Jie-Geng-Tang to disperse wind, clear the lungs, and relieve summer heat
Dry coating on the tongue, constipation, dry cough, dry skin, thirst, scanty and yellow urine	Dry heat: Qing-Zao-Jiu-Fei-Tang to clear dryness and lubricate the lungs

CHRONIC BRONCHITIS

The symptoms of chronic bronchitis are the same as in acute bronchitis, namely, cough, shortness of breath, and chest pain, except that in chronic bronchitis the symptoms are persistent and there is no fever. The persistence of symptoms in chronic bronchitis distinguishes it from chronic asthma, in which wheezing and breathlessness vary in severity from time to time.

SIGNS AND SYMPTOMS	SYNDROMES AND TREATMENT
Pale and swollen tongue with a greasy coating, coughing up phlegm easily, headache, pain in the chest, panting, insomnia, vomiting	Damp sputum: Er-Chen-Tang to strengthen the spleen, dry up dampness, transform sputum, and suppress cough
Red tongue with yellowish coating, coughing out yellow and sticky sputum in lumps, insomnia, stools with an offensive odor, vomiting, wheezing	Hot sputum: Qing-Qi-Hua-Tan-Wan to clear heat and transform sputum
Chronic backache, diarrhea, hair loss, ringing in the ears and deafness, seminal emission in men, toothache, whitish vaginal discharge, frequent miscarriage or infertility in women	Kidney deficiency: Du-Qi-Wan to tone the kidneys and increase the capacity of kidneys to absorb air, suppress cough, and transform sputum
Yellowish coating of the tongue, headache, dizziness, ringing in ears, jumpiness, red complexion, burning pain in the ribs, dry sensations in the mouth, bitter taste in the mouth, vomiting of blood or nosebleed in severe cases, yellowish urine, dry stools	Liver fire uprising: Xie-Bai-San to clear the lungs, calm the liver, and bring down fire

PNEUMONIA

Pneumonia is inflammation of the lungs caused by viruses or bacteria. Typical symptoms are fever, chills, shortness of breath, and cough with sputum or blood.

SIGNS AND SYMPTOMS	SYNDROMES AND TREATMENT
Red color of the tongue with yellow coating, coughing out yellow and sticky sputum, pain in the chest, pain in the throat, sputum with blood, craving for drink	Wind heat offending the lungs: Yin-Qiao-San to induce perspiration and expand lung energy
Coughing out copious yellow and sticky phlegm, chest pain	Pathogenic heat accumulated in the lungs: Ma-Xing-Gan-Shi-Tang to clear heat and expand the lungs
Fever particularly at night, slight thirst, coma, twitching, crimson tongue	Heat at the nutritive level: Qing-Ying-Tang to clear nutritive level, sedate heat, and open cavities

The cardiovascular system

HYPERTENSION

If you've been diagnosed with hypertension, it means you have high blood pressure, even when you are at rest. Hypertension is called the silent killer because you can have high blood pressure without knowing it. A person with hypertension may develop stroke or heart disease. When you have your blood pressure measured, the following table will help you assess the level of your blood pressure:

CLASSIFICATIONS	SYSTOLIC BLOOD PRESSURE	DIASTOLIC BLOOD PRESSURE
Normal	<130	<85
High normal	130–139	85–89
Mild	140–159	90–99
Moderate	160–179	100–109
Severe	180–209	110–119
Critical	>210	>120

SIGNS AND SYMPTOMS	SYNDROMES AND TREATMENT
Pale tongue with tooth marks visible, cold sensations in the body and cold limbs, dizziness, edema, fatigue, low voice, mental depression, ringing in ears, palpitations, underweight, perspiration easily triggered by movements	Simultaneous deficiency of yin and yang: Zhi-Gan-Cao-Tang to water yin and tone yang
Red and dry tongue, coughing out blood, excessive sex drive, hot sensations in the body, insomnia, jumpiness, night sweats, underweight	Yin deficiency with yang excess: Tian-Ma-Gou-Teng-Yin to nurture yin and weaken yang
Red tongue, bitter or sour taste in the mouth, blood in urine, dry throat, pain in the ribs, pink eyes with swelling, mental depression, spasms, twitching, vaginal discharge with fishy and offensive odor in women	Hot liver: Long-Dan-Xie-Gan-Tang to calm the liver and clear heat
Red tongue, dizziness, ringing in ears, hot sensations in the palms of hands and the soles of feet or numbness of limbs, difficulty in flexing and extending, jumpy muscles, seminal emission in men, scanty menstrual flow or suppression of menstruation in women	Yin deficiency of the liver and the kidneys: Shou-Wu-Tang to water kidneys and nourish liver

CORONARY HEART DISEASE, ANGINA PECTORIS, AND MYOCARDIAL INFARCTION

Coronary heart disease is a disease of the arteries that supply blood to the heart muscle; it causes damage to the heart or malfunction of the heart. The two most common forms of coronary heart disease are angina pectoris and myocardial infarction. Chest pain or a sensation of pressure in the chest is a sign of angina pectoris; the pressure is caused by insufficient oxygen carried to the heart muscle in the blood. Angina pectoris occurs particularly when the demand for oxygen is increased during intensive activities. Myocardial infarction occurs when part of the heart muscle dies suddenly, accompanied by severe heart pain in the center of the chest; this is commonly referred to as a heart attack. Other symptoms are shortness of breath, restlessness, and loss of consciousness. The diseases that contribute to myocardial infarction are hypertension, diabetes mellitus, and hyerlipidemias.

SIGNS AND SYMPTOMS	SYNDROMES AND TREATMENT
Red and shiny tongue with scanty coating on the tongue, and tooth marks visible, constipation, dizziness, dry cough with scanty sputum, dry mouth, dry stools, excessive perspiration, fatigue, frequent vomiting, hot sensations in the palms of hands and the soles of feet, light stomachache with swelling, palpitations, poor appetite, scanty urine, sore throat, thirst, fever in the afternoon	Yin and energy deficiency: this syndrome affects three internal organs in particular—lungs, spleen, and kidneys. Use Gua-Lou-Xie-Bai-Bai-Jiu-Tang with Dang-Gui-Bu-Xue-Tang to benefit energy, nurture yin, transform coagulations, and open up the passages of reticular meridians
Red tongue with white coating, abnormal perspiration, bleeding from gums, constipation, dizziness, dry and scanty stools, dry sensations in the mouth, dry throat, edema, excessive menstrual bleeding in women, fatigue, headache in the afternoon, night sweats, nosebleed, pain in the throat, insomnia, toothache	Yin deficiency: Gua-Lou-Xie-Bai-Bai-Jiu-Tang with Shou-Wu-Tang to nurture yin, tone kidneys, transform coagulation, and open the passages of reticular meridians
Pale tongue with tooth marks visible, cold sensations in the body and cold limbs, dizziness, edema, fatigue, low voice, mental depression, ringing in ears, palpitations, perspiration easily triggered by movement, underweight	Yin and yang both in deficiency simultaneously: Gua-Lou-Xie-Bai-Bai-Jiu-Tang with Zhi-Gan-Cao-Tang to tone both yin and yang, transform coagulation, and open up the affected meridians

CORONARY HEART DISEASE, ANGINA PECTORIS, AND MYOCARDIAL INFARCTION (continued)

SIGNS AND SYMPTOMS	SYNDROMES AND TREATMENT
Red and dry tongue, coughing up blood, excessive sex drive, hot sensations in the body, insomnia, jumpiness, night sweats, underweight, fever	Yin deficiency with yang excess: Gua-Lou-Xie-Bai-Bai-Jiu-Tang with Gou-Teng-Yin to nurture yin, oppress yang, transform coagulation, open up the affected meridians
Light-colored tongue with white coating, cold sensations, fatigue, frightened easily with rapid heartbeats, extremely cold hands and feet, pain in the chest and in the heart, palpitations with insecure feeling, profuse perspiration	Heart yang deficiency: Si-Ni-Tang with Sheng-Mai-San to warm yang, benefit energy, and restore the pulse to normal
Pale and swollen tongue with greasy coating, white and watery sputum that can be coughed up easily, dizziness, pain in the chest, panting, insomnia, suppression of menstruation in women, vomiting	Damp sputum: Ban-Xia-Bai-Zhu-Tian-Ma-Tang primarily to benefit energy and nourish yin, and secondarily to expel damp sputum

The urogenital system

ACUTE CHOLECYSTITIS AND GALLSTONE

Cholecystitis is inflammation of the gallbladder with severe abdominal pain on the right side of the abdomen just under the ribs, worsened by movements and sometimes accompanied by fever and jaundice. Acute cholecystitis is caused by the blockage of the cystic duct from the gallbladder by a gallstone; it may lead to chronic cholecystitis, in which the gallbladder walls thicken and the gallbladder itself shrinks until it ceases to store bile.

SIGNS AND SYMPTOMS	SYNDROMES AND TREATMENT
Swollen tongue, greasy and yellow coating on the tongue, abdominal pain, abnormal perspiration in hands and feet and the head, burning sensation and itch in the genitals, congested chest, diarrhea, low fever, thirst	Superficial damp-heat or damp-heat flowing downward: Long-Dan-Xie-Gan-Tang or Qing-Dan-Li-Shi-Tang to clear liver, reduce heat, and dry dampness
Gray coating on the tongue, complete suppression of urination, constant desire for drink but drinking only a little, pain in the throat with red swelling, vomiting that comes on rather suddenly	Excess heat: Long-Dan-Xie-Gan-Tang or Qing-Dan-Xie-Huo-Tang to clear liver, benefit gallbladder, promote bowel movements, and reduce heat
Blue-purple tongue with a glossy or white coating, abdominal pain, chest and ribs discomfort, chest pain, constipation, pain in inner part of stomach with pricking sensation and swelling, retention of urine, ringing in ears and deafness, stomachache, swelling and congestion after eating	Energy congestion: Long-Dan-Xie-Gan-Tang and Qing-Dan-Xing-Qi-Tang to clear liver, benefit gallbladder, promote bowel movements, and reduce heat

Urinary infections

Urinary infections include pyelonephritis or nephropyelitis (inflammation of the kidneys caused by a bacterial infection), cystitis or urocystitis (inflammation of the bladder caused by a bacterial infection), urethritis (inflammation of the urethra caused by a bacterial infection or other mechanisms). In traditional Chinese medicine, it is believed that the primary symptoms of this disease are frequent urination, urgency of urination, and pain on urination.

SIGNS AND SYMPTOMS	SYNDROMES AND TREATMENT
Red tongue with a yellowish-greasy coating, craving for cold drink, dry mouth, fever, frequent and urgent urination, burning sensation with urination, pain in the kidney zone, swelling and falling sensation of the lower abdomen or lower back pain	Damp heat: mostly seen in acute urinary infections or the acute stage of a chronic urinary infection. Use Dao-Chi-San, Ba-Zheng-San, or Long-Dan-Xie-Gan-Tang to clear heat and benefit dampness
White coating on the tongue, aversion to cold, cold limbs, fatigue, hot sensations in the palms of hands and the soles of feet, low-grade fever, pale complexion and pale lips, thin stools	Spleen-kidney deficiency: mostly seen in chronic urinary infections. Use Si-Jun-Zi-Tang with Ji-Sheng-Shen-Qi-Wan, Liu-Wei-Di-Huang-Wan, Zhi-Bai-Di-Huang-Wan, or Shen-Ling-Bai-Zhu-San to strengthen the spleen and tone the kidneys
Dark purple tongue or hemorrhages on the tongue, abdominal swelling, acute pain in the lower abdomen, burning sensation and pain on urination, congested chest, lump in the abdomen that stays in the same region, swollen pain in the chest with lumpy sensation and pricking pain	Energy stagnation and blood coagulation: Dan-Zhi-Xiao-Yao-San, Wu-Lin-San, or Gui-Zhi-Fu-Ling-Wan to disperse energy congestion and remove blood coagulation

ACUTE NEPHRITIS

Nephritis is inflammation of one or both kidneys; it may be acute or chronic. Nephritis includes two distinct forms. One is pyelonephritis, which is caused by a bacterial infection, often as a complication of cystitis, with such symptoms as a high fever, chills, and backache. The other is glomerulonephritis, which is an inflammation of the filtering units of the kidney called "glomeruli." It is a common cause of kidney failure.

SIGNS AND SYMPTOMS	SYNDROMES AND TREATMENT
Greasy or white coating on the tongue, chronic backache, diarrhea, fever that becomes more severe in the afternoon, headache with heavy sensations in the head, pain in all the joints, shifting pain, scanty urine	Wind dampness: Yue-Bi-Jia-Zhu-Tang to expel wind and promote water flow. This type of nephritis is characterized by puffiness
Red tongue with yellow coating, nosebleed, skin ulcer, abdominal pain that occurs at onset of periods in women, premature periods in women, vomiting of blood or nosebleed during periods	Hot blood: Xiao-Ji-Yin-Zi to clear heat and cool blood

CHRONIC NEPHRITIS

Chronic pyelonephritis often starts in childhood because of the backflow of urine from the bladder caused by a congenital abnormality of the valve. Two possible complications are hypertension and kidney failure. Glomerulonephritis, in which the glomeruli are damaged, may hamper the removal of waste products, salt, and water from the bloodstream, a condition that could lead to serious complications.

SIGNS AND SYMPTOMS	SYNDROMES AND TREATMENT
Greasy white coating on the tongue, absence of perspiration in hot weather, cold sensations in the lower abdomen and genitals, diarrhea, swollen limbs, pain in the body or the joints, period pain for women, scanty and clear urine, stomachache	Cold dampness: Si-Jun-Zi-Tang with Da-Huang-Fu-Zi-Tang to support yang and reduce dampness. This type of chronic nephritis falls within the category of uremia

CHRONIC NEPHRITIS (continued)

SIGNS AND SYMPTOMS	SYNDROMES AND TREATMENT
Red and dry tongue, coughing up blood, excessive sex drive, hot sensations in the body, insomnia, jumpiness, night sweats, underweight, fever	Yin deficiency with yang excess: Zuo-Gui-Wan with Liu-Wei-Di-Huang-Wan to water yin and oppress yang. This type of chronic nephritis is associated with hypertension
Light colored tongue with white coating, abdominal pain, indigestion, diarrhea, discharge of blood from the anus, discharge of copious sputum, edema, excessive menstrual bleeding in women, fatigue, weakness in the limbs and slightly cold, urge to lie down, poor appetite	Spleen deficiency: Si-Jun-Zi-Tang with Fang-Ji-Huang-Qi-Tang to strengthen the spleen
Red tongue with white or yellow coating, both eyes flickering or looking sideways or upward, dizziness with blurred vision, twitching and numbness in muscles	Liver wind: Ling-Yang-Gou-Teng-Tang with Da-Ding-Feng-Zhu to nurture yin, oppress yang, stop liver wind. This type of chronic nephritis falls within the category of uremia
Dark or pale tongue with thin white coating, dizziness, lower back pain, blurred vision, palpitations, shortness of breath	Spleen-kidney deficiency: Shi-Pi-Yin with Shen-Qi-Wan to warm and tone both the spleen and the kidneys

The blood and endocrine systems and the metabolism

DIABETES MELLITUS

Diabetes mellitus is characterized by increased sugar in the urine (glycosuria) and in the blood (hyperglycemia) caused by a disorder in the metabolizing of carbohydrates. Diabetes is normally diagnosed based on urine and blood tests.

1. Sugar in urine: A person with diabetes loses glucose proportionate to the severity of the disease and the intake of carbohydrates.

2. Sugar in blood: Blood sugar normally measures 60 to 100 mg/100 mL of blood; if it rises after a meal to as much as 150 mg/100 mL of blood, it might indicate diabetes mellitus. The blood sugar level in the early morning, at least eight hours after any previous meal, is normally 80 to 90 mg/100 mL. Any level higher than 120 mg/100 mL is considered diabetic. When a healthy person ingests one gram of glucose per kilogram of body weight, his or her blood glucose level rises from about 90 mg to about 140 mg/100 mL and falls back to below normal within two to three hours; thus, when blood sugar is raised above the normal range of 90 to 120 mg/100 mL of blood, the person is considered diabetic. Among the common symptoms are excessive urine production, excessive thirst, and increase in food intake, the appearance of boils and carbuncles, and weight loss.

SIGNS AND SYMPTOMS	SYNDROMES AND TREATMENT
Reddish tongue, slightly coated, coughing up blood, discharge of sticky sputum, dry sensations in the mouth, hoarseness, night sweats, hot sensations in the palms of hands and the soles of feet, insomnia	Lung yin deficiency: Bai-Hu-Jia-Ren-Shen-Tang or Xiao-Ke-Fang or Yu-Nu-Jian to nourish yin and clear heat
Reddish tongue, slightly coated, constipation, dry cough, dry lips, dry sensations in the mouth, low-grade fever, burning pain in stomach, vomiting or vomiting of blood, very poor appetite	Stomach yin deficiency: Tiao-Wei-Cheng-Qi-Tang or Xie-Xin-Tang to clear the stomach
Reddish tongue, sore pain across the loins, weak legs, dizziness, visual whirling sensations, ringing in ears, deafness, seminal emission in men, suppression of menstruation in women, infertility, night sweats, dry sensations in the mouth with no desire for drink	Yin deficiency of the kidneys: Liu-Wei-Di-Huang-Wan to water yin and tone kidneys

DIABETES MELLITUS (continued)

SIGNS AND SYMPTOMS	SYNDROMES AND TREATMENT
Swollen tongue with white or black coating on the tongue, chronic diarrhea, cold feet, cold loins and legs, cold sensations in the genitals or muscles, diarrhea before dawn, edema, fatigue, fear of cold, frequent urination at night, hair loss, pain in the loins, perspiration on the forehead, retention of urine, ringing in ears	Kidney yang deficiency: Shen-Qi-Wan to benefit the kidney and warm yang

SIMPLE GOITER AND HYPERTHYROIDISM

Simple goiter indicates a problem with the thyroid gland or with iodine intake. Hyperthyroidism refers to excessive secretion of the thyroid glands (thyroxine), which increases the basal-metabolic rate, causing an increased demand for food. The common symptoms are protrusion of the eyeballs, fine tremor of the extended fingers and tongue, nervousness, weight loss, excessive sweating, and increased heart rate.

SIGNS AND SYMPTOMS	SYNDROMES AND TREATMENT
Bluish tongue with white coating, cough, headache, desire for hot drink, menstrual flow light in color or morning sickness in women, feeling of a lump in the throat	Sputum congestion: Si-Hai-Shu-Yu-Wan to relax liver, relieve congestion, regulate energy, transform sputum
Headache, dizziness, ringing in ears, deafness, jumpiness, red complexion, burning pain in ribs, dry sensations in the mouth, bitter taste in the mouth, vomiting of blood or nosebleed in severe cases, yellowish urine, dry stools	Liver fire uprising: Long-Dan-Xie-Gan-Tang to clear liver and sedate fire

HYPOTHYROIDISM

Hypothyroidism refers to insufficient secretion by the thyroid glands of thyroxine, which reduces the metabolic rate. It may cause such symptoms as obesity, dry skin and hair, low blood pressure, slow pulse, and sluggishness.

SIGNS AND SYMPTOMS	SYNDROMES AND TREATMENT
Pale swollen tongue with greasy coating, watery sputum that can be coughed up easily, dizziness, pain in the chest, panting, insomnia, vomiting, suppression of menstruation in women	Damp sputum: Hai-Zao-Yu-Hu-Tang to transform sputum, benefit dampness, and transform coagulation
Bluish tongue with greasy coating, cough, headache, desire for hot drink, light color of menstrual flow or morning sickness in women, feeling of a lump in the throat	Sputum congestion: Si-Hai-Shu-Yu-Wan to relax liver, relieve congestion, regulate energy, and transform sputum
Reddish tongue with white coating, abnormal perspiration, bleeding from gums, constipation, dizziness, dry mouth and throat, pain in the throat, edema, fatigue, headache in the afternoon, night sweats, nosebleed, insomnia, toothache excessive menstrual bleeding in women	Yin deficiency involving the heart, the kidneys, and the spleen: Bu-Xin-Dan with Ban-Xia-Hou-Pu-Tang
Red tip of the tongue, dry stools, dry sensations in the mouth, low-grade fever, night sweats, palpitations and nervousness that get worse with movement, mental depression, insomnia with forgetfulness	Heart yin deficiency: Sheng-Mai-San with Er-Dong-Tang to nourish the heart, secure the spirit, water yin, and produce fluids
Headache, dizziness, ringing in ears, jumpiness, red complexion, burning pain in ribs, dry sensations in the mouth, bitter taste in the mouth, vomiting of blood or nosebleed in severe cases, yellowish urine, dry stools	Liver fire uprising: Long-Dan-Xie-Gan-Tang to clear liver and sedate fire

HYPOGLYCEMIA

Hypoglycemia refers to the deficiency of sugar in the blood, accompanied by increased insulin production. The common symptoms are acute fatigue, restlessness, malaise, marked irritability, mental disturbances, and hallucinations.

SIGNS AND SYMPTOMS	SYNDROMES AND TREATMENT
Pale swollen tongue with greasy coating, watery sputum that can be coughed up easily, dizziness, pain in the chest, panting, insomnia, vomiting, suppression of menstruation in women	Damp sputum: Tong-Jing-Zhu-Yu-Tang with Xiao-Yao-San to treat it
Purplish tongue or hemorrhagic spots on the tongue, abdominal swelling, congested chest, continual pain in one leg that gets worse on pressure, lump in the abdomen, pain in fixed regions that gets worse at night	Blood coagulation: Tong-Jing-Zhu-Yu-Tang to treat it

OSTEOPOROSIS

Osteoporosis is loss of protein matrix from bone, causing the bone to become less dense, more brittle and easily fractured, mostly as a result of aging. Women are more vulnerable to osteoporosis than men, particularly after menopause when the ovaries no longer produce estrogen hormones, which help maintain bone mass. Other causes of osteoporosis include calcium deficiency and removal of the ovaries. In traditional Chinese medicine, it is believed that this disease is mostly due to deficiencies in the spleen and kidneys and a reduction in blood and "pure essence" or *Jing*.

SIGNS AND SYMPTOMS	SYNDROMES AND TREATMENT
Pale tongue with white coating, pain in the affected region, excessive perspiration, fatigue, stomach discomfort, yellowish complexion	Blood deficiency and blood coagulation: Shen-Ling-Bai-Zhu-San with Dang-Gui-Si-Ni-Tang to strengthen the spleen and benefit energy

OSTEOPOROSIS (continued)

SIGNS AND SYMPTOMS	SYNDROMES AND TREATMENT
Red tongue, soreness across the loins, weak legs, dizziness, visual whirling sensations, ringing in ears, deafness, seminal emission in men, suppression of menstruation in women, infertility, night sweats, dry sensations in the mouth with no desire for drink	Kidney yin deficiency: Zhi-Bai-Di-Huang-Wan to reduce the kidney's yin and strengthen bone

HYPERLIPIDEMIA

Hyperlipidemia is a condition in which there is a high level of fats (lipids) in the blood. There are several forms of lipids, but the most common is cholesterol. Hyperlipidemia may be inherited or develop as a consequence of another disease such as diabetes, hypothyroidism, and kidney failure. The herbal formulas used to treat this disease are modern, because this disease was not recognized by traditional Chinese medicine until recently. I have therefore included the ingredients here.

A modern formula found to be effective for most syndromes of hyperlipidemia is called Dan-Tian-Jiang-Zhi-Wan: Chuan-xiong (rhizoma ligustici chuanxiong), 6 g; Dan-shen (radix salviae miltiorrhizae), 10 g; Dang-gui (radix angelicae sinensis), 11 g; He-shou-wu (radix polygoni multiflori), 15 g; Huang-jing (rhizoma polygonati), 15 g; Ren-shen (radix ginseng), 35 g; San-qi (radix notoginseng), 10 g; Ze-xie (rhizoma alismatis), 14 g.

SIGNS AND SYMPTOMS	SYNDROMES AND TREATMENT
Pale tongue with a thin coating, abdominal swelling, cold sensations, diarrhea with discharge of undigested foods, fatigue, poor appetite, weak limbs	For spleen kidney deficiency: Huang-Jing-Jiang-Zhi-Fang: He-shou-wu (radix polygoni multiflori), 12 g; Huang-jing (rhizoma polygonati), 20 g; Sang-ji-sheng (ramulus loranthi), 30 g, Shan-zha (fructus crataegi), 15 g

HYPERLIPIDEMIA (continued)

SIGNS AND SYMPTOMS	SYNDROMES AND TREATMENT
Pale swollen tongue with greasy coating on the tongue, watery sputum that can be coughed up easily, dizziness, pain in the chest, panting, insomnia, vomiting suppression of menstruation in women	For sputum dampness: Yin-Chen-Jiang-Zhi-Fang: Yin-chen (herba artemisiae scopariae), 15 g; Ze-xie (rhizoma alismatis), 15 g; Hu-zhang (rhizoma polygoni cuspidate), 15 g; He-ye (folium nelumbinis), 12 g; Gua-lou (fructus trichosanthis), 12 g; Chen-pi (pericarpium citri reticulatae), 6 g
Dark purplish tongue with a thick and greasy coating, chronic hoarseness, dry and sore throat, thickening of the vocal cord, vocal cord polyp, swelling with the feeling of a lump in the throat	For sputum congestion and blood coagulation: Tong-Mai-Jiang-Zhi-Fang: Chuan-xiong (rhizoma ligustici chuanxiong), 10 g; Hong-hua (flos carthami), Jiang-huang (rhizoma curcumae longae), 10 g; Xie-bai (bulbus allii macrostemi), 10 g; Chi-shao-yao (radix paeoniae rubra), 12 g; Gua-lou-pi (pericarpium trichosanthis), 12 g; Dan-shen (radix salviae miltiorrhizae), 15 g; Ge-gen (radix puerariae), 30 g
Thin coating on the tongue, abdominal pain, convulsions, numbness, stomachache, feeling of something stuck in the throat, vomiting of blood	For liver energy congestion: Shu-Gan-Jiang-Zhi-Fang: Chai-hu (radix bupleuri), 15 g; Jue-ming-zi (semen cassiae), 15 g; Ji-nei-jin (endothelium corneum/gigeriae galli), 12 g; Yu-jin (radix curcumae), 12 g; Chen-pi (pericarpium citri reticulatae), 6 g; Shan-zha (fructus crataegi), 10 g; Chuan-xiong (rhizoma ligustici chuanxiong), 10 g; He-ye (folium nelumbinis), 18 g

The nervous system

ARTHRITIS AND RHEUMATISM

Arthritis is inflammation of the joints, usually with pain and changes in structure. Rheumatism is a general term that refers to conditions characterized by soreness and stiffness of muscles, joints, and associated structures; it includes many forms of arthritis, such as infectious arthritis, rheumatoid arthritis, and gouty arthritis.

SIGNS AND SYMPTOMS	SYNDROMES AND TREATMENT
Pain in the joints all over the body that attacks suddenly, pain in the joints that shifts from one joint to another, shaking of the limbs and the entire body	Wind: Fang-Feng-Tang to expel wind and open the affected meridians
Absence of perspiration in hot weather, absence of thirst, abundant watering of eyes, severe pain in the joints	Cold: Wu-Tou-Tang or Wu-Ling-San or Xiao-Huo-Luo-Dan to disperse cold and remove dampness
Pain starts mostly in the lower regions of the body, pain always in same joints with heavy sensations of the body, pain in the loins as if sitting in water with heaviness in body	Dampness: Chu-Shi-Jian-Bi-Tang or Yi-Yi-Ren-Tang to remove dampness and activate the affected meridians

TRIGEMINAL NEURALGIA

Trigeminal neuralgia is also called "facial neuralgia" and *tic douloureux*; it refers to the neuralgia of the trigeminal nerve (the 5th cranial nerve), resulting in momentary (for as long as 20 seconds) pain that comes on in severe and sudden stabs and radiates along one of the three branches of the nerve.

SIGNS AND SYMPTOMS	SYNDROMES AND TREATMENT
Eyes cannot tolerate light and water abundantly	Liver wind heat: San-Huang-Xie-Xin-Tang to clear liver and stop wind
Profuse perspiration, spasmodic contraction of the anus, toothache	Bright yang meridian heat: the modern formula Xiong-Huang-San: Chuan-xiong (rhizoma ligustici chuanxiong) 10 g; Sheng-da-huang (radix et rhizoma rhei) 12 g; Mang-xiao (natrii sulfas) 10 g; Ban-lan-gen (radix isatidis) 10 g; Jin-yin-hua (flos lonicerae) 18 g; Zhi-qiao (fructus aurantii) 6 g; Huang-lian (rhizoma coptidis) 3 g; Jiang-chan (bombyx batryticatus) 6 g; Quan-xie (scorpio) 6 g
Hungry but with no appetite, pain triggered by eating and reduced by cold, ringing in ears and deafness, insomnia, thirst with no desire for drink	Sputum fire: Wen-Dan-Tang to transform sputum, clear heat, expel wind, and relieve pain
Red and dry tongue, coughing up blood, excessive sex drive, hot sensations in the body, insomnia, jumpiness, periodic and acute spasmodic pain, night sweats, underweight, seminal emission in men	Yin deficiency with yang excess: Da-Bu-Yin-Wan to water yin and subdue yang, stop wind, and relieve pain

TRIGEMINAL NEURALGIA (continued)

SIGNS AND SYMPTOMS	SYNDROMES AND TREATMENT
Bitter taste in the mouth, blood in urine, deafness, cloudy urine, dizziness, jumpiness, red eyes, rib pain, sudden onset of severe pain on the side of the head and face, watery eyes	Liver gallbladder excess fire: Long-Dan-Xie-Gan-Tang to expel wind, calm the liver, and clear bright yang heat
Purplish tongue or hemorrhagic spots on the tongue, acute onset of pain like electric shock, twitching of facial muscles in severe cases, pain in fixed regions that gets worse at night	Energy congestion and blood coagulation: Tong-Qiao-Huo-Xue-Tang to regulate energy, activate the blood, and expel wind

NEURASTHENIA

Neurasthenia is an ill-defined disease characterized by fatigue, weakness, headache, forgetfulness, anxiety, frustration, sweating, and insomnia.

SIGNS AND SYMPTOMS	SYNDROMES AND TREATMENT
Reddish tongue with white coating, abnormal perspiration, bleeding from gums, constipation, dizziness, dry and scanty stools, dry sensations in the mouth and throat, pain in the throat, edema, fatigue, headache in the afternoon, night sweats, nosebleed, insomnia, toothache, excessive menstrual bleeding in women	Yin deficiency, involving the heart, the kidneys, and the spleen: Bu-Xin-Dan with Ban-Xia-Hou-Pu-Tang to treat it
Red tongue with yellow coating, constipation, dry lips and mouth, thirst for cold drink, pain in the throat, acute fever, illness that attacks all of a sudden and changes rapidly, profuse perspiration, red complexion, red eyes, red urine	Excess fire or solid fire: Suan-Zao-Ren-Tang with Zhu-Sha-An-Shen-Wan to nourish yin, clear heat, calm liver, and secure the spirits

NEURASTHENIA (continued)

SIGNS AND SYMPTOMS	SYNDROMES AND TREATMENT
Red tongue with yellowish and greasy coating, cough, discharge of hard yellow sputum in lumps, cloudy and thin stools with an offensive odor, discharge of yellow, sticky sputum in lumps, dizziness with a desire to lie down, insomnia, blurred vision, vomiting, wheezing	Sputum heat and gallbladder energy deficiency: Wen-Dan-Tang to secure the spirits, relieve shock, transform sputum, and clear heat
Abdominal swelling, watery stools, fatigue, forgetfulness, impotence, nervousness, night sweats, palpitations, poor appetite, shortness of breath, insomnia, yellowish complexion	Heart spleen deficiency: Gui-Pi-Tang to nourish the heart, secure the spirits, strengthen the spleen, and benefit energy

SCIATICA

Sciatica is severe pain in the leg along the course of the sciatic nerve, which arises from the sacral plexus on either side, passing from the pelvis along the greater sciatic nerve and down to the back of the thigh and leg.

SIGNS AND SYMPTOMS	SYNDROMES AND TREATMENT
Pain increases at night, pain in one leg extending from the thigh toward the outside of the leg, pain intensified by cold, stabbing pain with burning sensations	Wind cold: Xiao-Huo-Luo-Dan to expel wind and disperse cold, increase dampness

SCIATICA (continued)

SIGNS AND SYMPTOMS	SYNDROMES AND TREATMENT
Red tongue, difficulty in both bowel movements and urination, dizziness, dry eyes, dry throat, fatigue, headache with pain in the bony ridge forming the eyebrow, lower back pain, night sweats, pain in one leg that gets worse on coughing or sneezing, insomnia with forgetfulness, seminal emission with dreams in men	Liver kidney yin deficiency: Du-Huo-Ji-Sheng-Tang to warm the kidneys and nourish the liver, disperse wind and cold, and expel dampness
Abdominal swelling, congested chest, continual pain in one leg that gets worse on pressure, pain in a fixed region that gets worse at night	Energy congestion and blood coagulation: Tao-Hong-Si-Wu-Tang to warm the meridians and activate the blood, transform coagulation, and relieve pain

CHAPTER 7
Diseases in Men

One should retain a smooth flow of energy and satisfy one's desires naturally; thus it is possible to obtain the satisfaction of every need.
—NEI JING

This chapter covers urinary disorders, diseases of the prostate, sexual dysfunction, and infertility in men.

Urinary disorders

In traditional Chinese medicine, urinary disorders are divided into two broad categories: urinary strains and suppression of urination. When a medical practitioner is treating the prostate, he will likely make references to these two categories. Urinary strains refer to disorders in which there is concern about passing urine, the quantity of the urine, and the quality of the urine.

URINARY STRAINS

SYNDROME	TYPES AND TREATMENT	URINATION	QUANTITY OF THE URINE	QUALITY OF THE URINE	OTHER SYMPTOMS
Hot urination syndrome	Use Ba-Zheng-San or Wu-Lin-San or Huang-Lian-Jie-Du-Tang with Wu-Wei-Xiao-Du-Yin to promote urination and remove dampness, clear heat, and detoxify	Burning sensation on urination	Normal	Red urine	Acute onset with fever, yellow and greasy coating on the tongue

URINARY STRAINS (continued)

SYNDROME	TYPES AND TREATMENT	URINATION	QUANTITY OF THE URINE	QUALITY OF THE URINE	OTHER SYMPTOMS
Bloody urination syndrome	Excessive type: Xiao-Ji-Yin-Zi to clear heat and promote urination, cool the blood, and stop bleeding	Painful and frequent	Normal	Blood in urine, red urine with dark bloody clots	Acute pain affecting the abdomen and navel, yellow coating on the tongue
	Deficient type: Di-Huang-Wan to water and tone kidney yin, clear heat, and stop bleeding	Painful	Normal	Blood in urine, light-red color	Lower back pain, light coating on the tongue
Energy congestion urination syndrome	Excessive type: Chen-Xiang-San to regulate energy and harmonize blood, relieve urinary strains, and promote urination		Dribbling of urine		Abdominal swelling and pain, white coating
	Deficient type: Bu-Zhong-Yi-Qi-Tang to tone the middle region and strengthen the spleen, and benefit energy	Frequent	Dribbling of urine	Clear urine	Abdominal swelling and pain, prolapse of the lower abdomen, pale complexion, pale tongue
Stony urination syndrome	Excessive type: Shi-Wei-San or Niao-Lu-Pai-Shi-Tang-Er-Hao-Fang or Ba-Zheng-San to remove sandy stones, relieve urinary strains, and promote urination	Difficult, with strong desire to pass urine, interrupted stream, acute pain on urination	Normal	Sandy stones in urine, blood in urine	Pricking pain on the urethra

URINARY STRAINS (continued)

SYNDROME	TYPES AND TREATMENT	URINATION	QUANTITY OF THE URINE	QUALITY OF THE URINE	OTHER SYMPTOMS
Stony urination syndrome (cont.)	Deficient type: Niao-Lu-Pai-Shi-Tang-San-Hao-Fang to benefit the kidneys and eliminate stones, sedate and tone simultaneously	Difficult, with strong desire to pass urine	Normal	Prolonged presence of sandy stones in urine	Pricking pain on urethra, dull pain in lower abdomen, burning sensations in "five hearts": palms of hands, soles of feet, and center of chest
Oily urination syndrome	Excessive type: Chen-Shi-Bei-Xie-Fen-Qing-Yin to clear heat and remove dampness, to clear the heart and promote energy flow	Difficult, with burning sensation on urination	Normal	Oily urine or milky urine, urine with floating oil, blood in urine	Red tongue, yellow and greasy coating
	Deficient type: Di-Huang-Wan with Jin-Suo-Gu-Jing-Wan to tone the kidneys and constrict urination	Difficult, with dull pain	Normal	Oily urine or milky urine	Recurrent onset, pale tongue, greasy coating

URINARY STRAINS (continued)

SYNDROME	TYPES AND TREATMENT	URINATION	QUANTITY OF THE URINE	QUALITY OF THE URINE	OTHER SYMPTOMS
Fatigued kidney syndrome	Kidney yin deficiency: Liu-Wei-Di-Huang-Wan	Frequent, burning sensation on urination	Normal		Chronic lumbago, hot sensation in five hearts, red tongue with scanty coating
	Kidney yang deficiency: Shen-Qi-Wan	Frequent	Long streams of urine		Aversion to cold, cold limbs
	Fatigued heart: Qing-Xin-Lian-Zi-Yin or with Dao-Chi-San	Difficult, with a desire to complete urination	Normal		Palpitations, shortness of breath, slight abdominal distention, fatigue, dry mouth and tongue, insomnia, red tip of tongue with thin white coating
	Fatigued spleen: Bu-Zhong-Yi-Qi-Tang with Di-Huang-Wan	Incomplete urination	Dribbling of urine		Symptoms intensified by fatigue

SUPPRESSION OF URINATION

SYNDROME	TYPES AND TREATMENT	URINATION	QUANTITY OF THE URINE	CONCURRENT SYMPTOMS
Excessive syndromes	Bladder damp heat: Ba-Zheng-San to clear heat and benefit dampness	Burning sensation on urination, difficult, painful on urination	Scanty urine	Greasy or yellowish coating on the tongue
	Hot lungs: Qing-Fei-Yin to clear lung heat and promote the urinary passage		Dribbling of urine or complete suppression	Dry and red tongue, bitter taste in the mouth, cough, dry throat, dry stools, chest pain, sore throat, yellow sputum
	Liver energy congestion: Chen-Xiang-San to smooth out the urinary mechanism and promote urination		Dribbling of urine or complete suppression	Red tongue with yellowish coating, pain in the chest, swelling and pain in the breast, jumpiness, or sensation of something in the throat
	Blood coagulation: Dai-Di-Dang-Wan to promote blood circulation and disperse energy congestion, promote urination		The streams of urine as small as lines, complete suppression of urination	Dark purple tongue with hemorrhagic spots, pain and swelling in the lower abdomen

SUPPRESSION OF URINATION (continued)

SYNDROME	TYPES AND TREATMENT	URINATION	QUANTITY OF THE URINE	CONCURRENT SYMPTOMS
Deficient syndromes	Falling of the middle energy: Bu-Zhong-Yi-Qi-Tang with Chun-Ze-Tang to elevate the clear and push down the turbid, transform energy and benefit water	Unable to pass urine due to lack of power	Scanty urine	Pale tongue with thin coating, shortness of breath, fatigue
	Yang deficiency of the kidneys: Ji-Sheng-Shen-Qi-Wan or Wen-Pi-Tang with Wu-Zhu-Yu-Tang to warm up yang and benefit energy, tone up the kidneys and promote urination		Scanty urine or complete suppression	Pale tongue with white coating, lumbago, cold sensations in the knees, decreased sexual desire, cold limbs
	Yin deficiency of the kidneys: Liu-Wei-Di-Huang-Wan with Zhu-Ling-Tang to water and tone kidney yin			Red tongue with clean or stripping coating, lower back pain, weak legs, dizziness, visual whirling sensations, ringing in ears, deafness, seminal emissions, night sweats

Diseases of the prostate

The prostate gland is located at the neck of the bladder, surrounding part of the urinary tract. This gland provides the seminal fluid that carries the reproductive sperm.

CHRONIC PROSTATITIS

Chronic prostatitis is inflammation of the prostate gland. It occurs most commonly in men between the ages of 20 and 40. Chronic prostatitis has a slow onset and progression; it may or may not be sexually transmitted. Chronic prostatitis is generally divided into chronic bacterial prostatitis and chronic nonbacterial prostatitis, but the two types display similar symptoms.

SIGNS AND SYMPTOMS	SYNDROMES AND TREATMENT
Discomfort and pain in the perineal area (between the anus and scrotum) and the lower abdomen and testes are the key symptoms, as well as lower back pain, blood in urine or in ejaculates, slight pain on urination	Energy congestion and blood coagulation: Qian-Lie-Xian-Tang to promote energy circulation and relieve coagulation
Frequent urination, burning pain in the penis, difficult urination, turbid discharge from the penis, pricking pain and itch, turbid and yellowish urine, constipation with dry stools, falling and swelling of the testes, red tongue with a thin or greasy coating	Damp heat obstruction: Ba-Zheng-San to clear heat and remove dampness
Lower back pain, weakened knees, dizziness, vertigo, ringing in the ears, insomnia, many dreams, seminal emissions, frequent erection, red tongue with scanty coating	Kidney yin deficiency with abundant fire: Zhi-Bai-Di-Huang-Wan or Da-Fen-Qing-Yin to water kidney yin and sedate fire

CHRONIC PROSTATITIS (continued)

SIGNS AND SYMPTOMS	SYNDROMES AND TREATMENT
Weakened knees, chills, cold limbs, impotence, seminal emissions, premature ejaculation, low spirits, pale complexion, turbid urine, pale and fat tongue with a thin layer of coating	Kidney yang deficiency: Gui-Fu-Di-Huang-Tang to warm kidney yang

ENLARGED PROSTATE GLAND

Enlargement of the prostate gland is common in men over the age of 50. The prostate gland surrounds a part of the urinary tract through which the urine is excreted. When the prostate gland is enlarged, it presses against the urinary tract and thus affects the normal passage of urine. When the urine is unable to pass through, it will accumulate in the bladder. If this continues, the urine will be forced back up into the kidneys, which may be damaged by the pressure of the contaminated urine to cause acute or chronic prostatitis. This obstruction to the bladder gives rise to a number of typical symptoms: frequent urination at night—more frequent when the disease gets more serious; a decrease in the quantity and force of the stream of urine; difficulty in starting urination; a constant desire to pass urine due to incomplete urination. An enlarged prostate is believed to be part of the normal aging process.

SIGNS AND SYMPTOMS	SYNDROMES AND TREATMENT
Dribbling of urine or difficult urination; dry throat and dry mouth; mental depression with a desire for drink; congested chest; shallow, rapid breathing; coughing and panting; red tongue	Hot lung: Qing-Fei-Yin to clear heat and benefit water, open and sedate lung energy
Frequent urination with dribbling of urine, burning and pain inside the penis, yellowish urine or blood in urine, thirst with no desire for drink, nervousness, difficult bowel movements or constipation, red tongue with yellowish or yellowish and greasy coating	Damp heat flowing downward: Dao-Chi-San with Ba-Zheng-San to clear heat and benefit dampness

ENLARGED PROSTATE GLAND (continued)

SIGNS AND SYMPTOMS	SYNDROMES AND TREATMENT
Scanty urine in yellow and red, inability to pass urine, dry throat and thirst, hot sensation on the palms of hands and soles of feet, ringing in the ears, dizziness, red complexion, mental depression with insomnia, distension in the lower abdomen, constipation with dry stools, red tongue with dryness, yellowish and greasy coating at the root of the tongue	Yin deficiency with abundant fire: Zhi-Bai-Di-Huang-Wan to water yin and bring down fire
Dribbling of urine, streams of urine as small as lines or complete suppression of urination, spastic sensation in the lower abdomen with swelling and pain, dark purple tongue with hemorrhagic spots on the tongue	Middle energy cave-in: Bu-Zhong-Yi-Qi-Tang with Chun-Ze-Tang to tone the middle region
A desire to pass urine but unable to do so, clear and whitish urine in small quantity, heaviness of the body with fatigue, shortness of breath and interrupted respiration, poor appetite, distension in the lower abdomen, pale and fat tongue with whitish coating	Kidney yang deficiency: Ji-Sheng-Shen-Qi-Wan to warm and tone kidney yang
Suppression of urination or dribbling of urine, too weak to urinate, pale complexion, poor spirits, lower back pain, chills, cold limbs, pale tongue with a thin layer of white coating	Liver energy congestion: Chai-Hu-Shu-Gan-Yin with Chen-Xiang-San to relax the liver and relieve congestion

ENLARGED PROSTATE GLAND (continued)

SIGNS AND SYMPTOMS	SYNDROMES AND TREATMENT
Sudden onset of suppression of urination or difficult urination, symptoms worsen with emotional stress, depression and jumpiness, swelling or pain in the abdominal region, a thin layer of yellowish or white coating on the tongue, red tongue	Energy congestion and blood coagulation: Dai-Di-Wan to disperse congestion and remove coagulation

PROSTATE CANCER

Prostate cancer is one of the most common cancers in men in middle age or in the elderly. Common symptoms are urination difficulty, poor flow of urine, and frequent urination. It is reported that when the formula Zhi-Bai-Di-Huang-Wan is used in combination with chemotherapy, the effects are remarkable.

SIGNS AND SYMPTOMS	SYNDROMES AND TREATMENT
Frequent urination, urgent urination, pain on urination, difficult urination, burning sensation on urination with red and short streams, back pain, distension in the lower abdomen, red tongue with yellowish and greasy coating	Damp heat congestion: Ba-Zheng-San to clear heat, benefit dampness, and promote urination
Dribbling of urine, interrupted urination, lumbago, pain and distension in the lower abdomen, dark-purple tongue with hemorrhagic spots	Energy congestion and blood coagulation: Ge-Xia-Zhu-Yu-Tang to transform coagulation and disperse congestion
Diminished urination or dribbling, powerless to push out urine, edema in the lower limbs, cold pain across the loins, weakened legs, pale complexion, poor spirits, dark color of the tongue with whitish coating	Kidney energy deficiency: Ji-Sheng-Shen-Qi-Wan to warm yang and benefit kidney energy

Sexual dysfunction

What is impotence and how do men become impotent? How quickly you have an erection often depends on your age. If you are in your twenties, you may have an erection within a few seconds. If you are in your sixties it might take five or ten minutes to get an erection, but this does not mean you are impotent. In addition, the time between erections also tends to increase with age. In some men aged 60 and over, it may take a whole week or longer to regain an erection, but again, that doesn't mean that they are impotent; it is simply a normal consequence of the aging process.

SIGNS AND SYMPTOMS	SYNDROMES AND TREATMENT
Cold sensations in the body, cold limbs, fatigue, dizziness, ringing in the ears, pale complexion. Aversion to cold and cold limbs are the focal symptoms in this classification	Kidney yang deficiency: Zan-Yu-Dan to tone the kidneys and warm up the kidneys and the penis
Low spirits with palpitations, insomnia, forgetfulness, many dreams, fatigue, poor appetite, withered and poor complexion, pale tongue, weak pulse. Palpitations, insomnia, fatigue, and poor appetite are the focal symptoms in this classification, because palpitations and insomnia are due to heart deficiency; fatigue and poor appetite are due to spleen deficiency	The heart and the spleen in deficiency: Gui-Pi-Tang to tone and benefit the heart and the spleen

SEXUAL DYSFUNCTION (continued)

SIGNS AND SYMPTOMS	SYNDROMES AND TREATMENT
Swelling of the scrotum, itch in the genital organs, weak legs, discharge of short streams of reddish urine, excessive stress, dizziness, yellowish and greasy coating on the tongue, itch in the inner thigh, discharge of reddish urine, yellowish and greasy coating on the tongue. The focus is on the liver, because it is due to heat accumulating in the liver that the patient displays many hot symptoms, such as reddish urine, swelling of the scrotum, and yellowish coating on the tongue	Damp heat flowing downward: Long-Dan-Xie-Gan-Tang to clear damp heat in the genital organs
Excessive stress, suspicious, jumpy, nervous, discomfort and pain in the chest and ribs, headache, dizziness, dry mouth and throat, fatigue, poor appetite, and emotional disturbances. The liver corresponds to anger in emotions; when the liver energy becomes congested, the patient will display emotional disorders, including anxiety, irritability, and stress	Liver energy congestion: Xiao-Yao-San to disperse the liver energy and relieve mental stress
Poor sexual drive, feeling pricking pain in the whole body, dark complexion, dark and purple color of the tongue with blood spots. When the arteries are clogged, it affects blood flow to the penis. For this reason, cholesterol and saturated fat are two contributing factors. This type of impotence is due to blood coagulation	Blood coagulation: Xue-Fu-Zhu-Yu-Tang to promote blood circulation and dissolve blood coagulation

SEXUAL DYSFUNCTION (continued)

SIGNS AND SYMPTOMS	SYNDROMES AND TREATMENT
Mental fatigue, low energy, dislike of talking, dizziness	Shock and fear harming the kidneys: Da-Bu-Yuan-Jian to tone the kidneys, relieve shock, and calm the spirits
Cold pain and swelling in the scrotum affecting the lower abdomen, absence of thirst, discharge of long streams of clear urine, aversion to cold, fever, headache, whitish coating on the tongue	Cold liver: Nuan-Gan-Jian to warm the liver, disperse cold, and relieve pain

FOOD CURES

BENEFICIAL FOODS FOR KIDNEY YANG DEFICIENCY: beef kidneys, chestnut, cinnamon, clove, clove oil, deer kidneys, dill seeds, fennel root, fennel seed, fenugreek seed (Oriental), lobster, oxtail, pistachio nut, raspberry, sheep or goat kidneys, shrimp, sparrow egg, star anise, strawberry, sword bean (jack bean).

BENEFICIAL FOODS FOR HEART AND SPLEEN DEFICIENCY: beef, beer, bird's nest, cherry, chicken, chicory, coconut, coffee, ginkgo leaf, ginseng, grape, honey, longan nuts, rock sugar, shiitake mushroom, tea, wheat.

BENEFICIAL FOODS FOR DAMP HEAT FLOWING DOWNWARD: azuki bean sprouts, buckwheat, cantaloupe, carp, celery root, Chinese cabbage, day lily, dried black soybean sprouts, eggplant, fig leaf, frog, hawthorn fruit, olive, soybean oil, soybean (yellow), squash flower, star fruit, wheat seedlings. *Foods to Avoid for Damp Heat Floating Downward:* alcohol, maltose, pork, sweet rice.

BENEFICIAL FOODS FOR LIVER ENERGY CONGESTION: beef, button mushroom; camphor mint, caraway seeds, cardamom seeds, carrots, chicken egg, chive, clam, dill seed, fennel seed, garlic, grapefruit, green onion (white part), hawthorn fruit, jasmine flower, kumquat, brown mustard, lichee nut and seed, longan seed, loquat seed, malt, marjoram, oregano, mussel, mustard seed, rapeseed (canola), red bean, roses, saffron, shiitake mushroom, spearmint, star anise, sweet basil, orange peel, tangerine orange and peel, turmeric, vinegar.

BENEFICIAL FOODS FOR BLOOD COAGULATION: brown sugar, camellia, cantaloupe, celery, chestnut, chicken blood, chickweed, chive, clam, coriander, crab, eggplant, fermented glutinous rice, ginger leaf, green onion (fresh juice and white part), hawthorn fruit, hemp, peach, radish, rapeseed (canola), rice (glutinous or sweet rice), soybean (black and yellow), sturgeon, sweet basil, tofu, turmeric, vinegar.

BENEFICIAL FOODS FOR SHOCK AND FEAR HARMING THE KIDNEYS: apple, beer, button mushroom, cantaloupe, cashew, celery, cinnamon, jackfruit, jasmine root, lily flower, longan, nutmeg, rice, rice bran, rosemary, watermelon, wheat, wheat seedlings.

BENEFICIAL FOODS FOR COLD LIVER: alcohol (moderate); cayenne pepper, chive, cinnamon, clove, coffee, garlic, ginger (fresh or dried), green onion, mustard seed, nutmeg, onion, pepper (black and white).

RECIPES FOR CURING IMPOTENCE

FOODS	RECIPES	SYNDROMES
Chicken liver	Rinse 2–3 chicken livers. Place on a plate with 25 g of honey and steam inside a pot. This is also good for night blindness and other vision problems. (Note: this recipe dates back to 1775.)	Good for cold liver
Lobster	Soak a 250 g lobster in 2 cups (500 mL) of wine for ten minutes. Fry the lobster and season to taste.	Good for kidney yang deficiency
Lamb kidney	Chop 3 lamb kidneys, 300 g mutton, and the white part of 1 green onion. Boil in water until well done. Use the broth to cook rice for meals. This is particularly good for impotence and weak legs associated with kidney deficiency.	
Chinese chive	Cut up 100 g Chinese chives and mix with 2 eggs. Add peanut oil and a little salt and fry. Eat at mealtime once a day for a week as a course of treatment.	
Mutton or lamb	Cut up 250 g mutton or lamb and peel 50 g garlic cloves. Boil the two ingredients in 3 cups (750 mL) water until cooked. Season with salt for consumption at mealtime, once a day. Repeat for 3 to 5 days.	

PREMATURE EJACULATION

Premature ejaculation refers to a man's inability to delay ejaculation long enough to induce orgasm in his sexual partner under normal circumstances. It is a common problem, especially for young males.

Under normal circumstances, a man should be able to maintain an erection for at least 10 to 20 minutes after penetration in order to be certain that the woman will be aroused and reach orgasm. Failure to last until a woman has reached orgasm is called premature ejaculation, which in many cases is due to a deficiency of kidney yin energy. If the yin energy is not strong enough to maintain the kidney fire, that fire is easily extinguished.

Why do men experience premature ejaculation? In seminal ejaculation, the semen is discharged by the male reproductive organs, and the mechanism that exercises control over the discharge is known as "the semen gate" in traditional Chinese medicine. When the semen gate is open, semen will pass through, resulting in seminal ejaculation; when the semen gate is closed, seminal ejaculation will not take place. If the semen gate remains open, semen will slide through freely; this is called "seminal sliding." In seminal sliding, the semen passes through slowly and freely, unlike in seminal ejaculation, in which the stream of semen is released suddenly. When a man complains of seminal sliding, his semen gate is open, but when he complains of premature ejaculation, his semen gate is loose. In either case, the semen gate must be fixed so that it can be properly opened and closed at will.

Quite a few Chinese herbal formulas, known as obstructive formulas, can be used to check premature ejaculation by blocking the movement of the semen gate so that it won't open so easily. Unlike yin tonics, which can slow down the movement of body fluids through their sticky nature, obstructive formulas can restrict the movement of body fluids. They can also roughen the surface of body tissues to make the movement of an object across the surface more difficult. To treat premature ejaculation, use Zhi-Bai-Di-Huang-Wan to delay ejaculation. When premature ejaculation is associated with erectile dysfunction, it should be treated as impotence.

Two typical foods that may be used to represent sliding nature and obstructive nature respectively are fresh honey and guava. Fresh honey has a sliding nature, but a green guava is so obstructive that one can develop constipation just by eating a few of them. When honey is cooked, it can become very sticky, which is why cooked honey is a yin tonic, with its original sliding nature disappearing. Thus when a person is suffering from diarrhea, fresh honey should be avoided but green guava may be recommended; when a person is suffering from constipation, green guava should be avoided, but fresh honey may be recommended. By the same token, when a man is suffering from premature ejaculation, foods or herbs with a sliding nature should be avoided, and foods or herbs with an obstructive nature may be recommended.

BENEFICIAL FOODS TO CHECK PREMATURE EJACULATION: chive, crabapple, black-eyed pea, fenugreek seed (Oriental), ginkgo (cooked), green guava, kelp, lotus fruit and seeds, mussel, palm root and seeds, peach (green and dried), plantain, pork kidney, rapeseed (canola), raspberry, string bean, walnut, yam.

RECIPE TO CHECK PREMATURE EJACULATION: Clean and chop 1 lamb kidney. Boil the kidney in water with 1 cup (250 mL) sweet, glutinous rice. Season to taste. This is particularly good for weak loins and knees associated with kidney deficiency.

NOCTURNAL EMISSIONS

Nocturnal emissions (commonly known as wet dreams) refer to ejaculation during sleep in the absence of intercourse. Seminal emissions may take place with or without erotic dreams and they are often accompanied by dizziness and backache. Sometimes, seminal emissions may take place during the daytime. An adolescent or an adult man who hasn't engaged in intercourse for a prolonged period may ejaculate once or twice a month; it is called overflowing of the semen and is considered normal.

Generally speaking, when seminal emission takes place with an erotic dream, it belongs to an excessive syndrome, which may include liver fire, damp heat in the liver meridian, or phlegm fire. When it is not accompanied by erotic dreams, it is a deficient syndrome, which may include kidney yin deficiency, kidney energy deficiency, no communication between the kidneys and the heart, or yin deficiency of the kidneys and the lungs combined. Without treatment, seminal emission may lead to sliding emission in which the semen simply slides through like running water.

SIGNS AND SYMPTOMS	SYNDROMES AND TREATMENT
Dizziness, ringing in the ears, lumbago, fatigue, skinniness, red tongue with dryness	Kidney yin deficiency: Zhi-Bai-Di-Huang-Wan to boost water to control fire
Poor complexion, poor spirits, aversion to chill, cold limbs, pale tongue with a layer of whitish coating	Kidney energy deficiency: Jin-Suo-Gu-Jing-Wan to tone the kidneys
Palpitation, fatigue, burning sensation on urination with a short and yellowish stream of urine, red tongue	No communication between the heart and the kidneys: Cai-Feng-Sui-Dan to clear the heart and water the kidneys
Seminal emission with an erotic dream, jumpiness, discomfort in the chest, red complexion, pink eyes, a bitter taste in the mouth, dry throat, short and reddish stream of urine, red tongue with a yellowish coating	Liver fire: Long-Dan-Xie-Gan-Tang to clear the liver and sedate fire
Frequent occurrences of seminal emission, semen in urine, a bitter taste in the mouth, thirst, burning sensation on urination with reddish urine, yellowish and greasy coating on the tongue	Damp heat in the liver meridian: Bei-Xie-Fen-Qing-Yin to clear heat and transform dampness
Frequent occurrences of seminal emission, congested chest, a bitter taste in the mouth, copious phlegm, difficult urination with reddish urine and a burning sensation, swelling of the lower abdomen and the genitals, yellowish and greasy coating on the tongue	Phlegm fire: Huang-Lian-Wen-Dan-Tang to transform phlegm and clear fire

COMMON RECIPES FOR SEMINAL EMISSIONS

FOODS	RECIPES	SYNDROMES
Sword bean	Clean 10 sword beans and cut a pork kidney into small pieces. Place the ingredients in a saucepan with 2 cups (500 mL) of water, and boil over low heat until water is reduced by half. Add a little salt to taste and serve. This is particularly good for chronic lower back pain, muscle pain across the loins, hard of hearing, and seminal emissions in men.	Good for kidney energy deficiency
Lotus seed	Boil the following ingredients in 1 to 2 cups (250–500 mL) of water until cooked: 10 g lotus seed, 30 g Job's tears, 15 g hyacinth bean. Divide into two portions for consumption at mealtime within one day. This is particularly good for kidney energy deficiency (seminal emission).	
Day lily	Boil 30 g lotus leaves and 10 g day lily in 1 cup (250 mL) of water until soft. Season to taste with sugar for consumption as one dose.	Good for phlegm fire

INFERTILITY

Male infertility may be due to four different syndromes, which are normally associated with either genetic deficiency or excessive sexual intercourse or masturbation. Modern medicine maintains that male fertility requires production of adequate quantities of viable, normal sperm by the testes, successful transport of sperm through the ducts, and successful delivery of the sperm in the vagina. Modern medicine also holds that male infertility is caused by any of the following three conditions: 1) lack of sperm in the semen or the absence of semen, 2) coagulation of the semen, or 3) abnormal semen. In traditional Chinese medicine, male infertility is caused by a decline in sexual energy with scanty semen, cold and diluted ejaculates, or premature ejaculation and impotence.

SIGNS AND SYMPTOMS	SYNDROMES AND TREATMENT
Kidney yang deficiency and kidney energy deficiency may cause a decline in sexual energy. When a man's sexual energy is in decline, either because of old age or illness or physical weakness, he will not be able to eject enough semen with a sufficiently strong force that it can reach far enough into the womb for conception. In the past when wealthy Chinese men had a dozen concubines, many men became infertile by the time they reached forty due to their sexual indulgence	A decline in sexual energy with scanty semen, which is normally due to kidney energy deficiency or kidney yang deficiency: Shen-Qi-Wan to tone the kidneys and improve sperm
The ejaculates are too cold and diluted, which means that they do not contain a sufficient amount of sperm to cause conception	Cold and diluted ejaculates due to deficient pure essence in the kidneys or kidney yang deficiency: Wu-Zi-Yan-Zong-Wan or Yang-Jing-Zhong-Yu-Tang to increase and improve semen production
When a man suffers from impotence or premature ejaculation, he may fail to send the sperm deep enough into the vagina	Premature ejaculation: Jin-Suo-Gu-Jing-Wan

SUMMARY OF MALE INFERTILITY AND HERBAL REMEDIES

SYNDROME	MODERN MEDICINE	CHINESE MEDICINE	HERBAL FORMULAS
Kidney yin deficiency	Lack of sperm in the semen; absence of semen	Inability to ejaculate, scanty semen	Wu-Zi-Yan-Zong-Wan with Gui-Lu-Er-Xian-Gao
Kidney yang deficiency	Lack of sperm in the semen; absence or non-emission of semen; abnormal semen	Cold and watery semen, scanty semen, a decline in sexual energy and scanty semen, impotence	Shen-Qi-Wan with Wu-Zi-Yan-Zong-Wan; or Wu-Zi-Bu-Shen-Wan with Zan-Yu-Dan
Kidney energy deficiency		Inability to ejaculate, a decline in sexual energy and scanty semen	You-Gui-Yin
Deficient pure essence in the kidneys		Cold and diluted ejaculates normally due to deficient pure essence in the kidneys or kidney yang deficiency	Wu-Zi-Yan-Zong-Wan
Relaxation of kidney energy		Premature ejaculation	Use Zan-Yu-Dan
Spleen deficiency	Lack of sperm in the semen	Scanty semen	Ren-Shen-Jian-Pi-Wan or Yi-Gong-San or Bu-Zhong-Yi-Qi-Tang
Blood coagulation	Lack of sperm in the semen, absence or non-emission of semen, abnormal semen	Inability to ejaculate, impotence	Xue-Fu-Zhu-Yu-Tang with Xiao-Yao-San or Dan-Shen-Yin or Tao-Hong-Si-Wu-Tang with Xue-Fu-Zhu-Yu-Tang
Damp heat in the liver meridian	Lack of sperm in the semen (spermacrasia), coagulation of the semen, absence or nonemission of semen. abnormal semen	Inability to ejaculate, scanty semen, premature ejaculation, impotence	Long-Dan-Xie-Gan-Tang, Bei-Xie-Fen-Qing-Yin, Qing-Re-Yu-Yin-Tang or Ba-Zheng-San
Yin deficiency with abundant fire	Coagulation of the semen	Inability to ejaculate, premature ejaculation	Zhi-Bai-Di-Huang-Wan or Da-Bu-Yin-Wan

SUMMARY OF MALE INFERTILITY AND HERBAL REMEDIES (continued)

SYNDROME	MODERN MEDICINE	CHINESE MEDICINE	HERBAL FORMULAS
Congestion and obstruction of phlegm dampness	Coagulation of the semen, abnormal semen	Obesity	Er-Chen-Tang with Shi-Xiao-San or Shao-Fu-Zhu-Yu-Tang
Energy deficiency		Inability to ejaculate	Gui-Pi-Tang
Blood deficiency	Absence or non-emission of semen		Shi-Quan-Da-Bu-Wan or Liu-Wei-Di-Huang-Wan
Deficient energy and blood	Abnormal semen		Dang-Gui-Bu-Xue-Tang or Ba-Zhen-Tang
Liver energy congestion	Abnormal semen	Inability to ejaculate, impotence	Xiao-Yao-San or Chai-Hu-Shu-Gan-San
Deficient heart and spleen		Premature ejaculation	Gui-Pi-Tang

RECIPE TO TREAT MALE INFERTILITY: Shrimp is particularly beneficial for kidney yang deficiency. Heat the fry pan. Pour in 1 teaspoonful of peanut oil and stir-fry 250 g shrimp until they are cooked. Add 100 g Chinese chives (chopped) and stir-fry again until the chives are cooked. Eat at mealtime.

CHAPTER 8

Treatment of Pregnancy Disorders

The mother and the fetus are in the same boat.
—GE ZHI YU LUN

Prenatal care

Prenatal care is the care of a pregnant woman and her unborn baby. It involves the general aspects of pregnancy, and includes daily routines, proper eating and exercise, and the emotional state of the pregnant woman.

Before we discuss pregnancy, however, let's look at what happens when a pregnancy terminates in miscarriage. Traditional Chinese medicine differentiates between two types of miscarriage. If miscarriage occurs during the first month of pregnancy the woman may not even be aware that fertilization has occurred. When a woman experiences more than one miscarriage during the first month of pregnancy, the womb may be damaged, leading to a pattern of habitual miscarriage. To avoid miscarriage in the first month, a woman who is trying to get pregnant should refrain from further intercourse for the remainder of what would be the menstrual cycle.

In traditional Chinese medicine, the duration of pregnancy is considered to be approximately 280 days, divided into ten lunar months

A Chinese classic on sexuality says, "A pregnant woman should not be in shock or fatigued or worried, nor should she eat raw foods, cold foods, sour foods, oily foods, or spicy foods in large quantities. Her mind should remain relaxed, listening to music and reading good books." Another Chinese physician named Zi-ming Chen (1190–1270) advised pregnant women by saying, "At long last, fertilization has taken place, which is indeed a great accomplishment. Now that the embryo has been formed, the mother should remember that the embryo in her womb will be affected by everything she does.... This is because the fetus inside the womb is affected by both the internal environments of the womb and the external environments in which the mother lives."

First of all, a pregnant woman should follow a daily routine. She should stay active but not allow herself to get exhausted. She should avoid strenuous activities such as carrying heavy loads or climbing steep hills. She should get enough sleep but not sleep too much. Lying down for extended periods of time can give rise to energy congestion, which can in turn contribute to a difficult labor.

The concept of a healthy pregnancy dates as far back as the publication of the *Nei Jing* in the third century BC. According to this medical classic, "When a pregnant woman is diseased, she will pass it on to her baby." In another classic, the author points out that King Zhou's mother was a virtuous lady with an excellent character. During her pregnancy, she "chose not to look at ugly things nor to hear abusive words, nor to make abusive remarks herself." Subsequently, she gave birth to a healthy baby with extraordinary intelligence. The baby grew up to become a great king who lived a very long life.

Emotion is considered a major topic in the discussion of prenatal care, because the pregnant woman's emotions provide the first stimulus to the fetus. The fetus also responds to the external environment in a very subtle way. If a pregnant woman feels upset or becomes highly emotional, either in extreme joy or anger, it may throw her internal organs into imbalance. Wan Quan, the author of the sixteenth-century medical classic *Wan Shi Nu Ke*, advises:

> When a pregnant woman is over-joyful, it will cause harm to the heart, because heart energy will disperse. When a pregnant woman is in excessive anger, it will cause harm to the liver, because liver energy will rush upward. When a pregnant woman is constantly in deep thought, it will cause harm to the spleen, because spleen energy will be congested. When a pregnant woman feels extremely sad, it will cause harm to the lung, because lung energy will be congested. When a pregnant woman is constantly in fear, it will cause harm to the kidney, because kidney energy will rush downward. After the energy of a pregnant mother is harmed, it will necessarily pass on to the fetus within her womb without exception. When energy of the pregnant woman is harmed, it may cause miscarriage. When energy of the fetus is harmed, it may impede the full growth of internal organs in the fetus, which may cause a series of disorders to the baby after it is born.

THE REGULATION OF SEXUAL DESIRES

Chinese medicine places taboos on intercourse at certain times in the reproductive cycle, such as during menstruation or pregnancy, or following childbirth. On those three occasions, a woman's physiology and psychology are undergoing drastic changes, her immunity is at a low level, and there is a vacuum in her body energy, which makes her most vulnerable to the attack of pathogens.

Sexual intercourse while the woman is menstruating is called "penis crashing into blood." It can cause damage to the woman's endometrium (lining of the uterus), infection, and other complications such as menstrual disorders and infertility.

Abstinence from sexual intercourse during certain stages of the pregnancy is an important measure to stabilize the embryo and prevent miscarriage. There is a general consensus among traditional Chinese doctors that sexual intercourse should not take place during the first two months and after the seventh month of pregnancy. The tiny meridian of the womb is connected to the kidney, which holds the fetus. Sexual intercourse during pregnancy will cause an excretion of yin energy in the pregnant woman, which should be used fully to nourish the fetus. In other words, her yin energy in the kidney will be spent on intercourse, reducing the capacity of the kidney to hold and nourish the fetus. This may cause an insecure fetus or miscarriage. It is only when the kidney is full of energy that the fetus will grow normally and the pregnant mother will be in good health. From the viewpoint of modern medicine, sexual intercourse during the first three months of pregnancy may cause pelvic congestion and uterus contraction due to sexual excitement and mechanical stimulation during intercourse, which may lead to miscarriage. Sexual intercourse after the seventh month of pregnancy may cause many complications, notably premature breaking of the waters, premature separation of placenta, or premature birth. Germs introduced to the vagina through intercourse may cause postnatal infection or fever.

AVOID DRINKING AND SMOKING

The spleen and the stomach are the sources of energy and blood. The growth and development of the fetus depend on the energy and blood of the mother. If a pregnant woman becomes intoxicated, the spleen and the stomach may be weakened, so that they cannot supply nourishment to the fetus. In addition, alcohol tends to produce dampness and heat in the body, which will pass to the fetus and cause fetal toxemia or fetal alcohol syndrome and muscular hypertrophy in the newborn baby. When a pregnant woman drinks too much, the alcohol in her body may transform into heat to cause fetal jaundice. In a Chinese medical text published in 1695, the author points out, "Fetal jaundice comes from the attack of damp heat on the womb, which is transmitted to the fetus. This is why a newborn baby looks yellowish in the face and eyes and throughout the body, with a high fever and constipation and passing red urine."

In another medical text published in 1742, the author concurs, saying, "Consumption of alcohol is very bad during pregnancy. The reason is that the fetus should absorb pure and peaceful energy from the mother. Alcohol is not only extremely hot, it also disturbs body energy and leaves it in chaos...."

Smoking, like drinking, is extremely harmful during pregnancy. The fetus is sensitive to the products of tobacco smoke in the blood of the pregnant woman. When a pregnant woman suffers from various symptoms caused by smoking, the baby's normal growth may be severely affected.

Women who smoke will be more likely to give birth to premature babies and unhealthy babies than non-smoking mothers will. Tobacco is pungent and hot, which may be transformed into fire fairly easily. When a pregnant woman smokes, the heat of tobacco may be transmitted to the womb to cause heat syndrome and other skin eruptions in the newborn baby.

MODERATE EXERCISE AND PROPER NUTRITION

A pregnant woman should strike a balance between work and leisure, particularly during the first and last three months of pregnancy. A healthy woman may participate in daily work, reducing her workload toward the last stage of pregnancy. She should do moderate exercise to promote energy and blood circulation and promote her own health and the health of the fetus, so that there will not be a miscarriage. A pregnant woman should refrain from doing strenuous work or taking hard exercise, which may contribute to miscarriage or premature birth or even premature separation of the placenta.

Foods are closely related to the growth of the fetus and that is why a pregnant woman should eat foods not only to meet her own needs, but also to meet the needs of the fetus. Foods considered especially beneficial during pregnancy are fish, egg, beans, celery, and orange. A pregnant woman should consume a wide variety of foods to create a balanced diet. She should not consume too much food with cold energy, such as salads, bamboo shoots, crab, grapefruit, and pineapple, because cold foods are harmful to the spleen and stomach. Greasy and fatty foods are difficult to digest and they are harmful to the spleen and may produce phlegm. Pungent and hot foods, such as spices, onion, and chive, may cause internal fire, which disturbs the fetus.

In the above-mentioned medical text from 1742, the author points out:

> *Infantile eczema attacks within one hundred days after birth; scaling and blisters occur on the head and in the face and cheeks that appear wide and round in different sizes. This is because the mother consumes an excessive quantity of pungent and hot foods during her pregnancy, which produces toxic heat in the womb and that accounts for the disease.*

Prenatal care month by month

From conception to the eighth week, the embryo develops into a fetus in the amniotic sac, surrounded by amniotic fluid in the uterus. The placenta, which is embedded in the uterus and attached to the fetus by the umbilical cord, provides nutrients to the fetus.

The ancient Chinese divided the baby's development into ten months during which special steps should be taken to nourish and protect the fetus on a monthly basis. In the Northern Qi Dynasty (550–577), a Chinese physician named Xu Zhi Cai published the *Monthly Schedules of Nourishing the Fetus*, in which he outlined a detailed program over the ten-month period. He points out that a pregnant woman "should regulate her eating habits, avoid getting too hungry or overeating, and should eat all the five flavors of food." After the seventh month of pregnancy, she should not eat too much salty food in order to prevent edema during pregnancy. The following is a summary of this classic schedule:

First month of pregnancy (1 to 4 weeks)
Development stage: The shaping month of the embryo.
Foods to eat or avoid: Eat polished cooked rice, sour foods, and barley; avoid pungent foods and fish.
Regulation of seven emotions: Avoid fear and shock. The pregnant woman's emotional state may have an impact on the embryo during this period.
Daily routine: A pregnant woman should refrain from doing hard labor, as well as engaging in sexual intercourse. She should sleep well and lead a quiet life.

Nourishing meridian: The liver meridian in particular should be nourished.

Treatment to avoid: Do not apply acupuncture and moxibustion on the liver meridian.

Second month of pregnancy (4 to 8 weeks)

Development stage: The basic shape of the embryo is formed.

Foods to eat or avoid: Avoid pungent foods and fish.

Regulation of seven emotions: Protect the body with great care and avoid shock.

Daily routine: Live in a quiet environment and avoid sex.

Nourishing meridian: The gallbladder meridian in particular should be nourished.

Treatment to avoid: Acupuncture and moxibustion should not be applied to the gallbladder meridian.

Third month of pregnancy (8 to 12 weeks)

Development stage: The fetus is still developing; it may easily be affected by the external environment.

Regulation of seven emotions: The image of anything bad viewed by the pregnant woman will be transferred to the fetus; avoid sadness, worry, and shock.

Adjustment of daily routine: Sit straight, be free from worry, control desires.

Nourishing meridian: The heart meridian in particular should be nourished.

Treatment to avoid: Acupuncture and moxibustion should not be applied to the heart meridian.

Fourth month of pregnancy (12 to 16 weeks)

Development stage: The fetus begins to receive water energy to fill up the blood vessels; the six bowels are formed.

Foods to eat or avoid: Eat rice and cake, fish, goose meat; eat moderately.

Adjustment of daily routine: Remain at rest and harmonious emotionally in order to strike a balance between energy and blood, facilitate eyesight and hearing, and promote energy flow in the meridians.

Nourishing meridian: Triple burning space meridian in particular should be nourished.

Treatment to avoid: Acupuncture and moxibustion should not be applied to the triple burning space meridian.

Fifth month of pregnancy (16 to 20 weeks)

Development stage: The fetus begins to fill energy and blood. The four limbs are complete.

Foods to eat or avoid: Eat rice, wheat and barley, pastry, beef, and lamb. Season food with five-spice powder, a Chinese seasoning made of star anise, cloves, cinnamon, fennel seed, and Szechwan peppercorns. Avoid extreme hunger, drinking too much water or eating too many dry foods. Refrain from applying heat to the body.

Regulation of seven emotions: Stay home and remain calm.

Adjustment of daily routine: Don't get too tired. Nurture body energy to secure the five viscera. Get up late, take a bath, and wash clothes.

Nourishing meridian: The spleen meridian in particular should be nourished.

Treatment to avoid: Acupuncture and moxibustion should not be applied to the spleen meridian.

Sixth month of pregnancy (20 to 24 weeks)

Development stage: The fetus begins to form the tendons and bones.

Foods to eat or avoid: Eat more meat to build up muscles and energy and strengthen the spine, refrain from overeating, season food with five-spice powder, and eat delicious foods.

Adjustment of daily routine: Try to be active. Don't stay indoors. Travel.

Nourishing meridian: The stomach meridian in particular should be nourished.

Treatment to avoid: Acupuncture and moxibustion should not be applied to the stomach meridian.

Seventh month of pregnancy (24 to 28 weeks)

Development stage: The fetus begins to form bones and marrow, and the skin and hair begin to grow.

Regulation of seven emotions: Don't shout or cry out loud.

Adjustment of daily routine: Be active and take a walk. Don't rest too much, but do some exercise to promote blood and energy circulation. Stay in a dry place. Focus on developing stomach energy and healthy teeth.

Nourishing meridian: The lung meridian in particular should be nourished.

Treatment to avoid: Acupuncture and moxibustion should not be applied to the lung meridian.

Eighth month of pregnancy (28 to 32 weeks)

Development stage: The fetus begins to develop skin; all nine cavities are built.

Foods to eat or avoid: Avoid dry foods.

Regulation of seven emotions: Stay calm and quiet. Don't move too much or perspire too much in order to keep the pores closed and the complexion healthy.

Adjustment of daily routine: Don't get too hungry or work too hard.

Nourishing meridian: The large intestine in particular should be nourished.

Treatment to avoid: Acupuncture and moxibustion should not be applied to the large intestine meridian.

Ninth month of pregnancy (32 to 36 weeks)

Development stage: The fetus begins to develop hair on the skin; the six bowels are complete.

Foods to eat or avoid: Drink sweet wine and eat sweet foods.

Adjustment of daily routine: Wear loose clothes to nourish the hair. Don't sit or lie on damp ground.

Nourishing meridian: The kidney meridian in particular should be nourished.

Treatment to avoid: Acupuncture and moxibustion should not be applied to the kidney meridian.

Tenth month of pregnancy (36 to 40 weeks)

Development stage: All meridians are built, the five viscera are complete, the six bowels are functioning, and the baby is ready to be born.

Adjustment of daily routine: Refrain from attending funerals. Prepare for labor. A Chinese doctor will advise the mother about delivery with six magic words: "Good sleep, pain tolerance, slow birth."

Treatment of prenatal disorders

Prenatal disorder symptoms will affect not only the pregnant woman's health, but also the fetus within her womb. In severe cases, the symptoms may cause miscarriage.

When prenatal symptoms are being treated, it is important to secure the fetus at the same time. To secure the fetus, tone the kidneys, strengthen the spleen, and promote energy circulation. If the pregnant woman is sick, the sickness should be treated accordingly.

Three rules apply if herbal remedies are used on a pregnant woman:

first, don't use herbs to induce perspiration; second, don't use herbs to induce bowel movements; third, don't use herbs to promote urination. If and when those herbs have to be used, they should be used with great care and in a small quantity for a short duration.

The most common prenatal symptoms are (1) morning sickness, (2) abdominal pain, (3) vaginal bleeding, (4) retarded growth of the fetus, (5) mental depression, (6) prenatal edema, (7) loss of voice, (8) cough, (9) prenatal urination disorders, and (10) prenatal suppression of urination.

1. MORNING SICKNESS

Typically, morning sickness begins around the sixth week of pregnancy, and symptoms peak during the eighth or ninth week and wane after the thirteenth week. The symptoms of morning sickness include nausea and vomiting, neither of which may require treatment. If symptoms are persistent and severe, they should be treated so that you can go through the pregnancy smoothly and avoid any damage to the kidneys and liver or to your unborn child.

The following are the three most common syndromes that account for most cases of morning sickness:

SPLEEN DEFICIENCY: The patient normally has a weak spleen and stomach. When she becomes pregnant, her yin blood flows downward to nourish the embryo, which creates a shortage of blood in the stomach. The shortage of blood creates a vacuum so that body energy rushes upward to the stomach to fill the gap, accounting for the nausea and vomiting in morning sickness.

DISHARMONY BETWEEN THE LIVER AND THE STOMACH: At the early stage of pregnancy, a woman's body uses blood from the liver, which creates a deficiency of blood in the liver. Since energy in the liver is active, it rushes upward to the stomach and causes nausea and vomiting. This phenomenon is called "liver energy offending the stomach" in traditional Chinese medicine.

DAMP PHLEGM OBSTRUCTING THE MIDDLE REGION: If a woman normally has an excess of damp phlegm in her body, the damp phlegm may be pushed up by fetal energy when she becomes pregnant to cause nausea and vomiting.

SYNDROME	DISTINCT SIGNS	GENERAL SIGNS	HERBAL FORMULA
Spleen deficiency	Vomiting of clear saliva, no appetite, no taste in the mouth	Vomiting right after eating, indigestion, sleepiness, fatigue	Xiang-Sha-Liu-Jun-Zi-Tang

FOOD CURES

SWEET RICE: Crush fresh ginger to produce 30 mL juice. Fry the juice with 250 g sweet rice until the rice cracks open. Grind the rice into a powder and store it in a jar. Take 20 g of the powder twice a day.

SUGAR CANE: Mix fresh sugar cane juice with a spoonful of fresh ginger juice. Drink it slowly at mealtimes, twice a day.

SYNDROME	DISTINCT SIGNS	GENERAL SIGNS	HERBAL FORMULA
Disharmony between the liver and the stomach	Vomiting of acid and bitter water	Congested chest, sighing, mental depression, bitter taste in the mouth, dizziness	Su-Ye-Huang-Lian-Tang to calm the liver and harmonize the stomach, reduce rising energy, and stop vomiting

FOOD CURES

GRAPEFRUIT PEEL: Cut up 15 to 20 g of grapefruit peel and boil them in 1 cup (250 mL) of water to drink like tea in one dose. Repeat as many days as necessary.

CHINESE CHIVE: Mix a tablespoonful of fresh Chinese chive juice with a tablespoonful of fresh ginger juice. Season it with a small amount of brown sugar to drink anytime.

SYNDROME	DISTINCT SIGNS	GENERAL SIGNS	HERBAL FORMULA
Damp phlegm obstructing the middle region	Nausea and vomiting of watery phlegm, dislike of drinking water	Full sensation in the chest with poor appetite, sticky and greasy sensation in the mouth	Xiao-Ban-Xia-Jia-Fu-Ling-Tang to dry up dampness and transform phlegm, harmonize the stomach, and relieve vomiting

FOOD CURE RECIPE

CHICKEN EGG: Put 60 mL of rice vinegar in a pan and bring to a boil. Add 30 g of white sugar, stirring to dissolve it. Crack an egg into the boiling vinegar and leave over heat until the egg is cooked. This mixture makes one dose. Take one dose a day for 3 to 5 days as a course of treatment.

2. ABDOMINAL PAIN

Prenatal abdominal pain is a recurrent pain in the lower abdomen with no vaginal bleeding. The Chinese call it "blockage of the womb." This symptom may be due to the following three syndromes; each of them should be treated differently.

BLOOD DEFICIENCY: The fetus is nourished by the mother's blood, and as the blood goes to the fetus, a shortage of blood is created in the lower abdomen. When blood is deficient in the lower abdomen, the lower abdomen cannot function as normal, which accounts for pain.

LIVER ENERGY CONGESTION: Energy is a yang force, which travels quickly along the liver meridian. When a pregnant woman is upset, abundant energy in the liver meridian may suddenly create congestion, just like a traffic jam. The energy congestion causes pain along the liver meridian, including the sides of the chest and sides of the lower abdomen.

DEFICIENCY AND COLDNESS: If a pregnant woman normally feels cold, it is because her yang energy is in short supply and her yin energy is excessive. When cold energy accumulates in her abdomen, she begins to experience abdominal pain, as cold energy will obstruct energy and blood circulation.

SYNDROME	DISTINCT SIGNS	GENERAL SIGNS	HERBAL FORMULA	FOOD CURES
Blood deficiency	Mild pain in the lower abdomen that continues on and on, which may be relieved by pressure of hand	Poor complexion, dizziness, fatigue, palpitations, poor sleep	Dang-Gui-Shao-Yao-San to nourish blood, secure the fetus, relieve the symptom, and lessen pain	Eat blood tonic foods, such as chicken soup, red bean and red date soup

SYNDROME	DISTINCT SIGNS	GENERAL SIGNS	HERBAL FORMULA	FOOD CURES
Liver energy congestion	Pain on the sides of the chest and the sides of the lower abdomen	Bad temper, poor spirits, and mental depression	Xiao-Yao-San to nourish blood and disperse liver energy congestion, regulate liver energy, and relieve pain	Drink a glass of orange juice to promote digestion
Deficiency and coldness	Cold pain in the lower abdomen that drags on and on; the pain may be reduced by heat	Cold sensations in the body and cold limbs, pale complexion	Jiao-Ai-Tang to warm yang energy and disperse cold, warm the womb, and relieve pain	Avoid cold foods, like salads and fruits, and also foods with cold energy, like clam. Drink a few cups of hot fresh ginger soup to warm the stomach

3. VAGINAL BLEEDING

In traditional Chinese medicine vaginal bleeding with the danger of miscarriage is called "leaking fetus" or "fetus motion," and spontaneous abortion is called "falling fetus" or "lesser birth" or "slippery fetus."

A pregnant woman may display intermittent vaginal bleeding, but it may also continue without stop. Vaginal bleeding during pregnancy is called "leaking fetus" in traditional Chinese medicine because bleeding is draining energy from the fetus. Sometimes, a pregnant woman might feel a sensation as if the fetus were falling down, followed by lower back pain and abdominal pain or discomfort or light bleeding from the vagina. This is called "fetus motion" or "insecure fetus." Vaginal bleeding and fetus motion are generally known as "threatened abortion" in Western medicine; these conditions often lead to miscarriage.

Natural loss of the fetus before the twelfth week of pregnancy, before the fetus is fully formed, is called "falling fetus." Loss of the fetus between the twelfth and twenty-eighth weeks of pregnancy after the fetus has been formed is called "lesser birth" or "half-birth." A woman who experiences three or more occurrences of falling fetus or lesser birth consecutively has carried a "slippery fetus" or a "multiple falling fetus," which is called "habitual spontaneous abortion" in Western medicine.

In general, falling fetus and lesser birth have come about as a result of leaking fetus and fetus motion, which is why leaking fetus, fetus motion, falling fetus, and lesser birth are manifested as different stages of the same disorder. The fetus is intact in leaking fetus and fetus motion and can still be saved. But in the cases of falling fetus and lesser birth, the fetus has been harmed or it has been expelled from the uterus.

The symptoms described above may be due to the following five syndromes, each of which should be treated differently.

KIDNEY ENERGY DEFICIENCY: A pregnant woman may have weak kidneys for several reasons: she has inherited the tendency from a parent; she has overindulged in sex; or a previous abortion or miscarriage has harmed the kidneys. It is more difficult for deficient kidneys to support the womb securely, a condition that accounts for fetus motion.

DEFICIENT ENERGY AND BLOOD: If a pregnant woman normally has a weak spleen and stomach, or if she has suffered a severe illness or a chronic consumptive disease, she will be more likely to experience a shortage of energy and blood to support the fetus. The Chinese think that energy in the womb carries the fetus, and blood in the womb nourishes the fetus. For that reason, deficient energy and blood may lead to vaginal bleeding and fetus motion.

HEAT IN BLOOD: The fetus requires blood for nourishment, so a pregnant woman's blood will be reduced and more energy than blood will be created in her womb. If, on top of that, a pregnant woman also experiences emotional disturbances, she will have energy congestion. When energy congestion is transformed into heat, bleeding and fetus motion result. And if a pregnant woman is in the habit of consuming spicy and hot foods, or if she is constantly under the influence of external heat, her blood may become heated gradually to cause bleeding.

BLOOD COAGULATION: A harmed fetus may obstruct blood circulation in the uterus. As bleeding continues and in increased quantity, the fetus may gradually leave the uterus, which accounts for the falling sensation and pain in the lower abdomen or partial expulsion of the fetus. Falling fetus and lesser birth may be due to this syndrome.

INJURY: A fall, a contusion, or excessive fatigue may cause harm to the womb so that it fails to carry and nourish the fetus, which is another cause of vaginal bleeding and fetus motion.

SYNDROME	DISTINCT SIGNS	GENERAL SIGNS	HERBAL FORMULAS	FOOD CURES
Kidney energy deficiency	Light bleeding from the vagina in pale or dark color	Lower back pain, falling sensation in the lower abdomen, dizziness, ringing in the ears, frequent urination	Shou-Tai-Wan or Bu-Shen-Gu-Chong-Wan to tone the kidneys and secure the fetus	Lotus seeds, raisins, shrimp, shiitake mushroom, raspberry, yam, walnut, strawberry, chicken
Deficient energy and blood	Light bleeding from the vagina in light-red color and thin in appearance	Fatigue with withered complexion	Ju-Yuan-Jian with Du-Shen-Tang to tone energy and blood and secure the fetus	Eat more foods beneficial to energy and blood, like chicken, red date, red bean. Eat one or two boiled eggs every day
Heat in blood	Slight bleeding from the vagina in fresh red color and sticky in appearanc	Mental depression, thirst, hot sensation in the palms of hands and the soles of feet, yellowish urine, constipation	Bao-Yin-Jian to clear heat, nourish blood, and secure the fetus	Drink more fresh fruit juice, like pear juice, grapefruit juice, and orange juice
Blood coagulation	Vaginal bleeding in large quantity within three months of conception, blood clots in bright red	Intermittent abdominal pain, swelling and falling sensation of the lower abdomen or overflowing of amniotic fluid, followed by increased bleeding	Sheng-Hua-Tang with Shi-Xiao-San to activate blood and transform coagulation, remove the fetus, and stop bleeding	Brown sugar, chestnut, eggplant, peach, papaya, radish, sweet rice, yellow and black soybean, to break up blood coagulation

SYNDROME	DISTINCT SIGNS	GENERAL SIGNS	HERBAL FORMULA	FOOD CURES
Injury	Pain and falling sensation in the lower abdomen	Lower back pain, light vaginal bleeding in red color	Sheng-Yu-Tang with Shou-Tai-Wan to benefit energy and harmonize blood, stop bleeding, and secure the fetus	Fresh fruit, pear, fresh lotus rhizome juice, sugar cane juice, to clear heat and produce fluids

4. RETARDED GROWTH OF THE FETUS

If, during the first four to five months of pregnancy, a pregnant woman's abdomen appears smaller than it should during this stage of pregnancy, but the fetus is alive and exhibiting slow growth, it is called retarded growth of the fetus or poor fetal growth (intrauterine growth retardation). The Chinese call it "withered and dry pregnancy" or "weak fetus." Babies suffering poor fetal growth are usually born underweight.

This symptom may arise from the following syndromes, each of which should be treated differently.

DEFICIENT ENERGY AND BLOOD: Poor fetal growth is usually due to failure of the placenta to provide adequate energy and blood to the fetus. Deficient energy and blood in the pregnant woman are the major causes of poor fetal growth.

SPLEEN AND KIDNEY YANG DEFICIENCY: If a pregnant woman has a poor appetite or if she suffers chronic diarrhea, her spleen may be weakened. The spleen takes charge of producing energy and blood in the body, which is why a pregnant woman with a weak spleen will not produce sufficient energy and blood to nourish the fetus. On the other hand, if a pregnant woman has genetically weak kidneys or if she has overindulged in sex, her kidneys may not support and nourish the fetus well.

SYNDROME	DISTINCT SIGNS	GENERAL SIGNS	HERBAL FORMULA	FOOD CURES
Deficient energy and blood	The abdomen appears smaller than usual after fifth month of pregnancy; skinny	In poor health, withered and yellowish complexion, dizziness, short breath	Ba-Zhen-Tang to tone energy and blood, so that they can be used to nourish the fetus	Ginseng, red date, bird's nest, spinach, peanut, duck, beef
Spleen and kidney yang deficiency	The abdomen appears smaller than expected for the length of pregnancy; watery stools	Abdominal swelling, lower back pain, poor appetite	Wen-Tu-Yu-Lin-Tang to tone the spleen and kidneys, nourish the fetus	Mussel, shiitake mushroom, chicken, lobster, mutton

5. MENTAL DEPRESSION

Depression in a woman during pregnancy ranges from being miserable and irritable to shock and being scared and angry. The Chinese call it "fetus depression." The symptoms may arise from the following two syndromes, each of which should be treated differently.

YIN DEFICIENCY: Yin deficiency may characterize a woman's physical condition before she is pregnant. And during pregnancy, her blood gathers to nourish the fetus, which may take a heavy toll on her blood condition. As blood is yin, blood deficiency may gradually drain off yin energy, leading to yin deficiency, which produces heat in the heart to cause depression.

PHLEGM FIRE: A woman may have copious phlegm in her system, and during pregnancy, excessive yang energy in her body may generate excessive heat, which burns the phlegm to become phlegm fire. When phlegm fire burns upward to the heart, it will cause depression.

SYNDROME	DISTINCT SIGNS	GENERAL SIGNS	HERBAL FORMULA	FOOD CURES
Yin deficiency	Being unhappy, palpitations, scary, unable to calm down	Hot sensations in the afternoon, hot sensations in the palms of hands and soles of feet, dry mouth and dry throat, red tongue	Ren-Shen-Mai-Dong-San to nourish yin and clear heat, secure the spirits, and relieve depression	Water chestnut, fresh lotus juice, lotus seeds. Avoid pungent and spicy foods, such as green onion, garlic, fresh ginger, cayenne pepper, tobacco, alcohol
Phlegm fire	Being insecure, unable to calm down, feeling depressed	Congested chest, nausea and vomiting, dizziness, red tongue, a layer of yellowish coating on the tongue	Zhu-Li-Tang to clear heat and remove phlegm, calm the heart and secure the spirits	Radish, agar, bamboo shoot. Avoid pungent and spicy foods, such as green onion, garlic, fresh ginger, cayenne pepper, tobacco, alcohol

6. PRENATAL EDEMA

A woman may display puffiness in her face and eyes and limbs during pregnancy. If the puffiness fails to disappear after a full night of rest, it is called prenatal edema or "swelling of the fetus" according to the Chinese. Edema that occurs only in the legs toward the end of pregnancy with no other discomfort is considered normal and should disappear by itself after delivery without treatment. This symptom may arise from the following three syndromes, each of which should be treated differently.

SPLEEN YANG DEFICIENCY: The spleen loves dryness, and a deficient spleen is most vulnerable to an attack of dampness. When this happens, water may invade the face and eyes and four limbs to cause puffiness, which could affect the whole body in severe cases.

KIDNEY DEFICIENCY: The kidneys are unable to warm the spleen in the upper region and warm the bladder in the lower region when they are deficient. The spleen and the bladder are important organs in promoting water metabolism, and when they are incapable of performing, water will accumulate in the body to cause edema.

ENERGY CONGESTION: When energy circulation slows down, it will impede water metabolism. As water has a tendency to flow downward, edema will start in the feet and cause difficulty in walking. As energy circulation slows down, no yang energy is moving to the head, causing a heavy sensation in the head due to shortage of yang energy.

SYNDROME	DISTINCT SIGNS	GENERAL SIGNS	HERBAL FORMULA
Spleen yang deficiency	Edema in the face, or the whole body, manifested as a slight depression in the skin when finger pressure is applied	Light yellowish skin, shortness of breath, too lazy to talk due to fatigue, poor appetite, watery stools	Bai-Zhu-San to strengthen the spleen and promote water flow

FOOD CURES

CARP: Clean the fish. Cut a 100 g wax gourd into pieces. Boil the fish and wax gourd in water until cooked. Season the broth with salt and oil. Eat the fish and wax gourd and drink the soup once a day for a week.

PEANUTS: Soak 150 g of peanuts in warm water to remove coating. Remove seeds from 12 red dates. Dice 40 g of garlic. Put half a teaspoonful of peanut oil into a frying pan set on high heat. Add the garlic when the frying pan is hot. Quickly add the peanuts, red dates, and a glass of water, and boil until cooked. Divide the mixture into two portions for consumption at mealtimes. Repeat for one week.

AZUKI BEANS: Steam a gold carp with 90 g of azuki beans in 2 cups (500 mL) water over high heat until cooked. Consume once a day for 5 to 7 days consecutively.

SYNDROME	DISTINCT SIGNS	GENERAL SIGNS	HERBAL FORMULA
Kidney deficiency	Edema, particularly the lower limbs manifested as a deep depression in the skin when finger pressure is applied	Puffy face and eyes and the four limbs, short of breath, palpitation, dizziness, ringing in the ears, cold limbs, chills, lower back pain, pale tongue	Zhen-Wu-Tang to warm yang energy and promote urination

SYNDROME	DISTINCT SIGNS	GENERAL SIGNS	HERBAL FORMULA
Energy congestion	Edema starts from feet and it is manifested as a depression in the skin when finger pressure is applied, and the depression rebounds to its original contour when pressure is released	No change in skin color, dizziness and headache with a heavy sensation in the head	Tian-Xian-Teng-San to regulate energy and promote its circulation

FOOD CURES

BLACK SOYBEAN: Dice 30 g of garlic. Put the garlic, 100 g of soybeans, and 30 g of red dates in a frying pan. Add 1 cup (250 mL) of water and boil until cooked. Season the mixture with brown sugar and divide it into two portions for consumption at mealtimes for a week.

AZUKI BEANS: Put 100 g of azuki beans, 100 g of black soybeans, and 50 g of mung beans in a frying pan. Add 2 cups (500 mL) of water and boil until beans are soft. Season the mixture with white sugar and divide it into three portions for consumption at mealtimes for a week.

7. LOSS OF VOICE

A pregnant woman may experience hoarseness or inability to talk in the later stages of pregnancy, most often in the ninth month of pregnancy. This symptom may arise from kidney yin deficiency because the fetus has grown big and obstructs the kidneys; kidney yin becomes incapable of flowing to the woman's throat for nourishment. On top of that, a pregnant woman needs more yin blood to nourish the fetus, which creates a likelihood of kidney yin deficiency. If there are no other complications, this symptom will disappear after delivery without treatment.

HERBAL CURES	Liu-Wei-Di-Huang-Wan to water the kidney to benefit yin energy
FOOD CURES	Drink honey water to nourish yin energy and moisten the lungs. Avoid consumption of pungent and hot foods, which can consume yin energy

8. COUGH

A pregnant woman may cough continually without stop, often accompanied by hot sensations in the five centers (in the center of the chest, palms of the hands, and soles of the feet). The Chinese call it "cough of the fetus." This symptom may arise from the following two syndromes, each of which should be treated differently.

YIN DEFICIENCY AND DRY LUNGS: Yin deficiency means that there is not sufficient yin to go to the throat, so that the throat will be dry; it also means that the lungs will also be short of yin energy, which results in dry lungs.

PHLEGM FIRE DISTURBING THE LUNGS: Yin deficiency may give rise to yang excess, which in turn heats up the phlegm in the lungs to disturb them. When the phlegm becomes hot, it will be sticky and difficult to cough up.

SYNDROME	DISTINCT SIGNS	GENERAL SIGNS	HERBAL FORMULA	FOOD CURES
Yin deficiency and dry lungs	Dry cough or coughing up blood	Persistent cough during pregnancy, dry throat, red tongue with a scanty coating	Bai-He-Gu-Jin-Tang to nourish the yin and lubricate the lungs, stop cough and secure the fetus	Pear, honey, white fungus, white sugar, apple, lemon
Phlegm fire disturbing the lungs	Coughing up sticky and yellowish phlegm with difficulty	Persistent cough, red complexion, dry throat, and red tongue with a layer of yellowish and greasy coating on the tongue	Xiao-Xian-Xiong-Tang to clear heat, transform phlegm, and relieve cough	Radish, seaweed, kelp, pear, sugar cane

9. PRENATAL URINATION DISORDERS

A pregnant woman may experience frequent urination, urgent urination, pain on urination, urination difficulty, or spasm in the lower abdomen, all of which are classified under urinary disorders in traditional Chinese medicine. This symptom may be attributed to a malfunctioning of the bladder to obstruct the free passage of urine. The symptoms may arise from the following three syndromes, each of which should be treated differently.

HEART FIRE FLAMING UPWARD: When yin deficiency gives rise to heart fire, it will flame upward to the face. The heat may be transmitted to the bladder through the small intestine, because the heart and the small intestine form a yin–yang relationship. When the bladder gets too hot, its function of excreting urine may be disordered.

DAMP HEAT FLOWING DOWNWARD: In the syndrome of heart fire flaming upward, fire from the heart flames upward to the face, and it also flows downward to the bladder through the small intestine. But fire from the heart may focus on flowing downward to the bladder, in which case the forceful heat may get mixed with the water in the bladder to cause burning pain on urination.

YIN DEFICIENCY: Kidney yin deficiency may create kidney yang excess, which generates heat in the bladder.

SYNDROME	DISTINCT SIGNS	GENERAL SIGNS	HERBAL FORMULA	FOOD CURES
Heart fire flaming upward	Pain on urination, urination difficulty, yellowish urine	Frequent urination, red complexion, mental depression, ulcers on the tongue, cankers in the mouth	Dao-Chi-San to sedate fire in the heart, nourish yin, and lubricate dryness	Green tea, white fungus, lotus seed, asparagus, banana, cucumber, bamboo shoots

FOOD CURE RECIPE

RICE: Boil 100 g of rice in water. Add the white heads of 3 green onions when the rice is almost cooked and continue to boil for 1 minute. Divide into two doses for consumption on an empty stomach. This is particularly good for suppression of urination due to a damaged bladder.

SYNDROME	DISTINCT SIGNS	GENERAL SIGNS	HERBAL FORMULA	FOOD CURES
Phlegm fire disturbing the lungs	Burning pain on urination, yellowish and reddish urine	No thirst, red tongue with a layer of yellowish and greasy coating on the tongue	Jia-Wei-Wu-Lin-San to clear heat and benefit dampness, promote urination and relieve pain	Radish, watermelon, cucumber, mung bean, common carp

FOOD CURE RECIPE

BROAD BEAN: Grind 50 g of dried broad beans and boil the powder with 6 g of tea leaves. Drink it like tea. This is particularly good for suppression of urination during pregnancy due to lung energy deficiency.

SYNDROME	DISTINCT SIGNS	GENERAL SIGNS	HERBAL FORMULA	FOOD CURES
Yin deficiency	Frequent urination with discharge of scanty urine in yellowish color, burning sensation and pricking pain on urination	Hot sensations in the palms of hands and soles of feet, dry stools, poor sleep, red tongue with a layer of yellowish coating on the tongue	Zhi-Bai-Di-Huang-Wan to water the yin and lubricate dryness, clear heat, and promote urination	Pork, royal jelly, wax gourd, white fungus, day lily, longan nuts, white sugar

SYNDROME	DISTINCT SIGNS	GENERAL SIGNS	HERBAL FORMULA	FOOD CURES
Energy deficiency	Suppression of urination or frequent urination with scanty urine, acute pain in the lower abdomen	Fatigue, short breath, pale complexion, pale tongue with a thin layer of white coating	Yi-Qi-Dao-Niao-Tang to increase kidney energy and promote urination	Ginseng soup or ginseng powder
Kidney deficiency	Suppression of urination or frequent urination with scanty urine, swelling and pain in the lower abdomen	Chills and cold limbs, lower back pain, pale tongue with a thin layer of moist coating on the tongue	Shen-Qi-Wan to warm the kidneys and boost yang energy to promote urination.	Mutton, beef

FOOD CURE RECIPE

CHINESE CHIVES: Cut up 150 g of Chinese chives and fry it in a frying pan. Add 250 g fresh shrimps to the frying pan and fry until cooked. Season to taste with salt and black pepper. This is particularly good for suppression of urination or incontinence of urination during pregnancy due to kidney deficiency.

10. PRENATAL URINATION SUPPRESSION

A pregnant woman may experience suppression of urination, acute pain in the lower abdomen, and mental depression with little sleep. This symptom is called the "turning of the fetus" in traditional Chinese medicine, because the falling of the fetus, which exerts pressure on the bladder to block its passage, causes it. This symptom may arise from the following two syndromes, each of which should be treated differently.

ENERGY DEFICIENCY: A woman with energy deficiency before pregnancy may find herself having more difficulty in supporting the fetus as it grows bigger and bigger. Consequently, the fetus falls on the bladder to cause suppression of urination.

KIDNEY DEFICIENCY: The kidneys support the fetus within the womb during pregnancy. A woman with kidney deficiency may not be able to support the fetus with her kidney energy, so that the fetus falls on the bladder to cause suppression of urination.

CHAPTER 9

Postnatal Care and Treatment of Disorders

It is fairly easy for a new mother to get sick; it is very difficult for her to recover from an illness. —CHAN YUN JI

A new mother needs special care for a period of two months or longer after giving birth. The postnatal period is divided into three periods: the new period, the interim period, and the last period. The new period lasts seven days after birth, the interim period lasts thirty days after birth, and the final period lasts sixty days after birth. The genital organs in a new mother need six to eight weeks to recuperate from the impact of childbirth.

As a new mother, you should be careful about daily routines. Be moderately active and avoid heavy work. During the new period, you should be resting most of the time; during the interim period, you should refrain from doing housework; and during the last period, you should refrain from doing heavy work. You should also eat carefully and try to eat more foods that are easily digestible, neither too hot nor too cold in food energy. If you eat too many cold or hot foods, spicy foods or greasy foods, and fried foods, it may disturb your blood circulation or dry up the yin energy in your body. It is also important to regulate your emotions, as extreme emotions may easily disturb your energy and blood. As a new mother, you should not engage in sexual intercourse in most cases until the last period is over, or within one hundred days from birth in other cases.

Postnatal disorders are illustrated in the following chart with reference to their causes and mechanisms:

CAUSES			MECHANISMS	DISORDER
Yin blood suffers a drastic setback, vital energy is grossly lessened by labor	Deficient yin blood or energy	Excessive consumption of spicy and dried foods, which causes harm to yin energy; or excessive fatigue causes harm to the spleen	Deprivation of blood causes damage to body fluids, dispersing of yang energy, deficient energy and blood, contaminated blood running wild	Three basic postnatal disorders (spasms, fainting, and difficult bowel movements), night sweats, persistent discharge, suppression of urination, excessive perspiration, excessive milk secretion, dizziness
Prone to blood coagulation	Existing energy congestion and blood coagulation	Seven emotions become extreme, and attack by pathogens	Internal obstruction of blood coagulation	Abdominal pain, dizziness, fever, persistent discharge, three basic postnatal invading disorders by contaminated blood (lung disorder, stomach disorder, heart disorder)
Grossly deficient joints caused by labor	Chronic weakness	Attack of pathogens, irregular eating, careless sexual intercourse	Loss of balance between energy and blood, loss of balance in the functions of internal organs	Postnatal fever and pain in the body

Treatment of postnatal disorders

Right after delivery, you will feel physically weak and suffer from low immunity. Consequently, you need a fairly long period of recuperation. The Chinese medical classic *Bei Ji Qian Jin Yao Fang,* published in 652, contains this statement: "A new mother can have sexual intercourse only one hundred days after delivery. Otherwise, it will make her weak and vulnerable to all kinds of disease during her entire life. A mother who is frequently ill and feels cold sensations below her umbilicus may have had sexual intercourse shortly after delivery." In addition, a nursing mother should not have sexual intercourse too frequently, as it may deprive her of energy and blood, compromising her milk supply.

The symptoms that you can expect to experience for six to eight weeks after delivery are called "postnatal symptoms." The uterus and genitals will return to their natural pre-pregnancy state during this period. The most common postnatal symptoms are 1) dizziness and fainting, 2) abdominal pain, 3) persistent discharge, 4) difficult bowel movements, 5) fever, 6) urination disorders, 7) perspiration and night sweats, 8) postnatal pain in the body, 9) lack of lactation, or 10) spontaneous and persistent lactation.

DIZZINESS AND FAINTING

After delivery, you may suddenly feel dizzy and unable to stand, or you may experience a congested sensation below the heart, nausea and vomiting, presence of phlegm in the throat, mental depression, nervousness, lockjaw, and fainting in severe cases. The symptoms may arise from the following two syndromes, each of which should be treated differently:

BLOOD DEFICIENCY WITH A SUDDEN FALL IN ENERGY: If you suffer blood deficiency before pregnancy, your blood may become even more deficient after childbirth due to loss of blood during delivery. After a heavy loss of blood, your energy may collapse as a result.

BLOOD COAGULATION WITH ENERGY UPRISING: You are most vulnerable to disease during or shortly after delivery. If cold energy attacks you during this period, it may cause blood coagulation. Coagulated blood may push energy to move upward, which is called uprising energy, and this may lead to dizziness and fainting.

SYNDROME	DISTINCT SIGNS	GENERAL SIGNS	HERBAL FORMULA	FOOD CURES
Blood deficiency with a sudden fall in energy	Sudden dizziness, pale complexion	Palpitation, fainting, cold limbs, cold sweats, closed eyes, open mouth	Du-Shen-Tang to benefit energy and fix prostration	Chicken soup, longan, red bean, red date

DIZZINESS AND FAINTING (continued)

SYNDROME	DISTINCT SIGNS	GENERAL SIGNS	HERBAL FORMULA	FOOD CURES
Blood coagulation with energy uprising	Prior to fainting, there is pain in the lower abdomen that intensifies on pressure	No discharge after delivery or scanty discharge, congestion below the heart, short breath, presence of phlegm in the throat, fainting with lockjaw	Duo-Ming-San to promote blood circulation and dissolve blood coagulation	Black fungus, cayenne pepper, coriander, garlic, ginger (fresh), tea, tofu, water chestnut

ABDOMINAL PAIN

Afterpains arise from contractions of the uterus that may continue after delivery; these pains are normal, because the uterus continues to shrink, as it should. Afterpains usually disappear within three to five days after delivery. If the pain continues or intensifies over an extended period, you are experiencing a condition called postnatal abdominal pain. This symptom may arise from the following two syndromes; each of them should be treated differently:

BLOOD DEFICIENCY: The vigorous meridian and the conception meridian become empty after loss of blood during delivery, leading to blood deficiency.

BLOOD COAGULATION: You are most vulnerable to attack of disease during or shortly after delivery. If cold energy attacks you during this period, it may cause blood to coagulate. Or if you are affected by anger, it may cause liver energy to congest, leading to blood coagulation.

SYNDROME	DISTINCT SIGNS	GENERAL SIGNS	HERBAL FORMULA	FOOD CURES
Blood deficiency	Mild abdominal pain, love of warmth and massage	Scanty discharge, pale in color, dizziness, ringing in the ears, palpitation, excessive perspiration, dry stools, pale tongue with a thin layer of coating	Chang-Ning-Tang to tone up energy and blood and relieve pain	Red date and longan soup. In cases of constipation, drink honey water

FOOD CURE RECIPE

Chop up 15 g of fresh ginger and 400 g of mutton. Put them in a pot, and add 2 cups (500 mL) of water. Put the pot in a steamer and set over medium heat until cooked. Divide the mixture into three portions for consumption at mealtime once a day for three consecutive days. Repeat for a six-day course of treatment.

SYNDROME	DISTINCT SIGNS	GENERAL SIGNS	HERBAL FORMULA	FOOD CURES
Blood coagulation	Pricking pain in the lower abdomen that may be intensified by pressure	Scanty discharge after delivery, dark in color, pain on the sides of the chest, cold limbs, dark color of tongue with bloody spots on the sides	Sheng-Hua-Tang to activate blood and remove coagulation, disperse cold, and relieve pain	Fresh ginger with brown sugar soup

FOOD CURE RECIPE

Put 50 g of dried hawthorn fruit in a fry pan, add 1 cup (250 mL) of water, and cook over low heat for 20 minutes. Add 30 g of brown sugar and bring the mixture to a boil. Drink it hot once a day for a week.

Persistent Discharge

Lochia is the discharge of blood and fragments of uterine lining from the vagina; this discharge usually ceases within six weeks after delivery. The discharge is bright red for the first three or four days, then becomes light red and within two weeks becomes yellowish or whitish. If the discharge continues beyond the normal period of six weeks, it is called persistent discharge of lochia and should be treated. This symptom may arise from the following three syndromes; each of them should be treated differently:

ENERGY DEFICIENCY: When a woman suffers an excessive loss of blood during delivery, she is more likely to develop blood deficiency, which will cause energy deficiency. In addition, excessive fatigue may cause harm to the spleen, possibly leading to blood deficiency because the spleen produces blood. Lochia is part of blood, and energy controls blood. When energy is deficient, it fails to control blood, so the discharge continues without stop.

HEAT IN THE BLOOD: When a woman suffers yin deficiency before pregnancy, she is more likely to continue the yin deficiency because she will lose blood during delivery. Yin deficiency may cause heat in blood. Consuming too much hot and spicy food during pregnancy may also generate heat in blood. Constant anger during pregnancy may generate heat in the liver, which stores blood. Heat in blood will cause bleeding, which intensifies the discharge.

BLOOD COAGULATION: A woman's meridians are almost empty after delivery, making her more vulnerable to the attack of external cold, which will cause blood coagulation. Premature consumption of constrictive herbs or other drugs may also cause blood coagulation.

SYNDROME	DISTINCT SIGNS	GENERAL SIGNS	HERBAL FORMULA	FOOD CURES
Energy deficiency	Continual discharge in large quantities and in pale color	Pale complexion, dizziness, fatigue, shortness of breath, feeling of emptiness in the lower abdomen, fat tongue	Bu-Zhong-Yi-Qi-Tang to tone energy and constrict blood	Beef, bird's nest, chicken, ginseng, red date, rice (sweet), sugar (brown and rock), tofu

SYNDROME	DISTINCT SIGNS	GENERAL SIGNS	HERBAL FORMULA	FOOD CURES
Heat in blood	Continual discharge is purple or bright red, sticky and offensive	Pain in the lower abdomen, mental depression, dry mouth and dry throat, red tongue with a layer of dry coating	Bao-Yin-Jian to nourish the yin and clear heat, stabilize the vigorous meridian, and stop the bleeding	Fresh lotus, pear, sugar cane, watermelon. Avoid pungent and spicy foods
Blood coagulation	Continual discharge in small quantities and dark in color with clots	Pain in the lower abdomen that intensifies on pressure, bloody spots on the sides and tip of the tongue	Sheng-Hua-Tang to activate blood and transform coagulation, stabilize the vigorous meridian, and stop bleeding	Drink fresh ginger with brown sugar soup

POSTNATAL DIFFICULT BOWEL MOVEMENTS

This symptom may be caused by a blood deficiency. When a woman suffers blood deficiency before pregnancy, loss of blood during delivery may intensify it. Blood deficiency may dry up intestinal fluids, which in turn causes dryness in the intestines.

SYNDROME	DISTINCT SIGNS	GENERAL SIGNS	HERBAL FORMULA	FOOD CURES
Blood deficiency	Difficult bowel movements, dry stools	Dry skin, no abdominal swelling or pain, normal appetite, withered and yellowish complexion, pale tongue with a thin layer of coating	Si-Wu-Tang to nourish blood and lubricate dryness	Honey, vegetables, fresh fruits; drink more water. Avoid pungent and spicy foods and alcohol

FOOD CURE RECIPES

WALNUT: Grind 30 g of walnuts and 30 g of black sesame seeds into a powder. Mix the powder with 100 g sweet, glutinous rice and boil it in 2 cups (500 mL) of water until the rice becomes very soft. Eat it in one day in one dose. This is particularly good for constipation due to blood deficiency.

POTATO: Peel and cut up 500 g of potatoes and boil them in 2 cups (500 mL) of water until soft. Add 1 teaspoon of brown sugar. Eat the mixture before bedtime. This is particularly good for constipation due to blood deficiency.

SESAME OIL: Mix 2 tablespoons of sesame oil with 3 tablespoons of honey and boil over low heat for five minutes. Take half a tablespoon each time, twice daily. This is particularly good for constipation due to blood deficiency.

POSTNATAL FEVER

Postnatal fever refers to the continual fever that fails to reduce or a high fever, with other complications. A woman may display low fever within one to two days after delivery without complications; this fever, called "physiological fever," not postnatal fever, will clear up without treatment. A woman may display low fever during the lactation period three to four days after delivery (the Chinese call it "steaming milk"), but this will disappear by itself without treatment; it is not postnatal fever. In general, to be considered a postnatal fever, your temperature must be over 38°C and last over two to three days, or it must be a continual low fever. This symptom may arise from any of the following four syndromes; each of them should be treated differently:

TOXIC PATHOGEN ATTACK: When a woman is harmed by delivery or suffers severe bleeding during delivery, her body energy becomes incapable of defending itself against toxic pathogen attack (bacterial or viral infections in Western medicine). A vigorous struggle between body energy and toxic pathogens gives rise to high fever.

BLOOD COAGULATION: Incomplete discharge of lochia after delivery causes blood coagulation. When blood coagulation occurs, it may cause a loss of balance between body surface and the internal region, which accounts for fever.

ATTACK OF EXTERNAL PATHOGENS: A woman is vulnerable to the attack of external pathogens, such as wind and cold, which can cause fever, as in the common cold.

BLOOD DEFICIENCY: Under normal circumstances, energy and blood work together. When a woman suffers blood deficiency after delivery, her blood becomes incapable of supporting energy so that energy and blood separate from each other, with energy floating to the superficial region. Floating energy is manifested as low fever and perspiration.

SYNDROME	DISTINCT SIGNS	GENERAL SIGNS	HERBAL FORMULA	FOOD CURES
Toxic pathogen attack	High fever that fails to go down, aversion to cold, chills	Pain in the lower abdomen that intensifies on pressure, discharge dark in color with an offensive smell, thirst, scanty urine in red color, constipation, red color of the tongue with a layer of yellowish coating on the tongue	Jie-Du-Huo-Xue-Tang to clear heat and counteract toxic effects, cool blood, and transform coagulation	Fresh juice, watermelon, lotus juice
Blood coagulation	Alternating chills and fever after delivery	Scanty discharge dark in color with clots, pain in the lower abdomen that intensifies on pressure, and thirst with no desire for drink	Sheng-Hua-Tang to activate blood and transform coagulation	Drink fresh ginger with brown sugar soup

SYNDROME	DISTINCT SIGNS	GENERAL SIGNS	HERBAL FORMULAS	FOOD CURES
Attack of external pathogens	Fever with aversion to cold	Headache, pain in the body, nasal congestion and discharge, cough, no perspiration, a thin layer of white coating on the tongue	Use Jing-Fang-Si-Wu-Tang to support body energy and relax, expel external pathogens, and expand the lungs	Drink fresh ginger with brown sugar soup, hot rice soup to induce perspiration
Blood deficiency	Heavy loss of blood after delivery, low fever that drags on	Perspiration, dizziness, palpitations, insomnia, numbness of the limbs	Use Ba-Zhen-Tang to tone energy and blood, nourish yin, and clear heat	Chicken soup, white fungus. Avoid pungent and spicy foods

POSTNATAL URINATION DISORDERS

Urination difficulties are quite common in women after delivery. Suppression of urination, frequent urination, and incontinence fall within the category of postnatal urination disorders.

A woman should be able to urinate within six to eight hours after delivery. If she is able to urinate but displays difficulty doing so or if she cannot pass urine at all, she is suffering from postnatal suppression of urination. By contrast, a woman who urinates more than twenty times a day after delivery, with no pain or urgency, is suffering from frequent urination. In more extreme cases, a woman may temporarily lose control over urination after delivery.

Although the above three types of urination disorders are manifested in different sets of symptoms, they are all connected with delivery and attributable to the same syndromes. The disorders all arise because the bladder is unable to function properly, but they are also associated with the kidneys and the lungs. The kidneys are in control of the bladder and the lungs are in communication with the bladder to regulate water metabolism. The symptoms may arise from the following three syndromes; each of them should be treated differently:

LUNG ENERGY DEFICIENCY: The lungs push water downward to the bladder for excretion. Lung energy deficiency makes the lungs unable to control the function of pushing water downward, and the bladder is affected, causing urination disorders.

KIDNEY ENERGY DEFICIENCY: The kidneys are in control of the bladder, which controls urination. When there is energy deficiency, the kidneys are unable to control the bladder, affecting the bladder and causing urination disorders.

DAMAGED BLADDER: The bladder may be damaged during delivery, resulting in the involuntary escape of urine.

SYNDROME	DISTINCT SIGNS	GENERAL SIGNS	HERBAL FORMULA	FOOD CURES
Lung energy deficiency	Suppression of urination or frequent urination, tense sensation in the lower abdomen	Clear, whitish urine, pale complexion, fatigue, low voice, pale tongue with tooth marks on the tongue	Bu-Zhong-Yi-Qi-Tang to tone energy of the lungs	Beef, chicken, longan, pork, shiitake mushroom, shrimp
Kidney energy deficiency	Suppression of urination or frequent urination, escape of urine, swelling and pain in the lower abdomen	Lower back pain, dark complexion, pale tongue	Shen-Qi-Wan to tone kidney energy and warm yang energy of the kidneys	Chicken, raspberry, shrimp, shiitake mushroom, strawberry, walnut, yam

FOOD CURE RECIPE

Steam 3 g of cinnamon bark with 2 chicken livers for consumption as one dose. This is particularly good for urination disorders due to kidney energy deficiency.

SYNDROME	DISTINCT SIGNS	GENERAL SIGNS	HERBAL FORMULA	FOOD CURES
Damaged bladder	Continual involuntary escape of urine after delivery, which may be mixed with silky blood	Normal tongue	Huang-Qi-Dang-Gui-San to tone energy and strengthen the bladder	Beef, brown sugar, celery, chicken, corn, lemon, mung bean

FOOD CURE RECIPE

Boil 60 g of mung beans, 100 g of pork liver, and 1 cup (250 mL) of rice together in water and season to taste. This is particularly good for edema and decreased urination associated with liver deficiency and damaged bladder. (This recipe was first created in 1578.)

POSTNATAL SWEATING AND NIGHT SWEATS

A woman may sweat a lot after delivery, particularly while moving around during the daytime. Or, a woman may sweat a lot at night, but sweating stops after waking up, a condition known as "night sweats." Sweating during the daytime arises from energy deficiency; night sweats arise from yin deficiency.

ENERGY DEFICIENCY: A woman may experience energy deficiency after delivery, because pregnancy normally takes a heavy toll. If there is insufficient energy, body fluids will be easily excreted and sweating will occur.

YIN DEFICIENCY: A woman may suffer from yin deficiency before pregnancy. She loses blood during delivery, which further contributes to her existing condition. At night, yin energy floats to the body surface, which accounts for night sweats.

SYNDROME	DISTINCT SIGNS	GENERAL SIGNS	HERBAL FORMULAS	FOOD CURES
Energy deficiency	Excessive sweating during the daytime, which gets worse while working or moving	Aversion to wind, pale complexion, shortness of breath, too tired even to talk, pale tongue with a thin coating	Huang-Qi-Tang or Yu-Ping-Feng-San to tone the energy and close the pores	Chicken, longan, red date, rice (sweet), soybean (black), wheat

FOOD CURE RECIPE

Boil 60 g of wheat in water. Discard the wheat, retaining the broth to use as soup. Add 100 g of rice and 5 red dates to the soup and boil it again. Divide it into two equal portions to eat at mealtime; continue until the condition improves.

SYNDROME	DISTINCT SIGNS	GENERAL SIGNS	HERBAL FORMULAS	FOOD CURES
Yin deficiency	Night sweats, no sweating while awake	Complexion bright red, dizziness, ringing in the ears, dry mouth, dry throat, hot sensations in "five centers" (in the center of the chest, palms of hands and soles of feet), the tongue is deep red	Sheng-Mai-San with Zhi-Han-San to rejuvenate the yin and benefit energy, produce fluids, and check night sweats	Black fungus, chicken, day lily, duck, green turtle, wax gourd, white fungus

FOOD CURE RECIPE

Boil 60 g of pork liver and 1 chicken egg or 250 g of spinach together. This is particularly good for blurred vision, night blindness, and corneal disorders.

POSTNATAL PAIN IN THE BODY

A woman may experience postnatal pain in her body, most notably in her limbs, a numbness, and a heaviness, with no local swelling or burning sensation. If, however, the pain extends beyond six or seven weeks after delivery, it does not fall within this category. This symptom may arise from the following four syndromes; each of them should be treated differently:

BLOOD DEFICIENCY: If a woman suffers blood deficiency before pregnancy, her blood may become even more deficient after delivery due to loss of blood during delivery. After heavy loss of blood, her blood will not be abundant enough to nourish the four limbs, the body, the meridians, and the joints, causing numbness and pain to those regions.

EXTERNAL ATTACK OF WIND AND COLD: A woman is more vulnerable to an external attack after delivery, when her body is weak. If she is exposed to wind and cold and dampness at this juncture, the external pathogens may penetrate into her body to cause pain in various regions.

KIDNEY DEFICIENCY: The kidneys nourish bones and marrow, and they support the fetus within the womb during pregnancy. When the kidneys are deficient, the bones and marrow may become weak and painful.

BLOOD COAGULATION: Blood coagulation may occur after delivery; it causes pain in different regions, depending on the location of coagulated blood.

SYNDROME	DISTINCT SIGNS	GENERAL SIGNS	HERBAL FORMULA	FOOD CURES
Blood deficiency	Pain all over the body after delivery, numbness of limbs, pain in the limbs	Withered complexion, dizziness, palpitation, the tongue is light red with scanty coating on the tongue	Huang-Qi-Gui-Zhi-Wu-Wu-Tang to nourish blood and benefit energy, warm the meridians, and promote circulation	Azuki bean soup, longan, lotus soup, pork liver, red date
External attack of wind, cold, and dampness	Stiff joints and pain in fixed joints are due to dampness, wandering pain throughout the body is due to wind, and severe pain is due to cold	Walking difficulty, pain relieved by warmness, pale tongue, and a thin layer of coating on the tongue	Du-Huo-Ji-Sheng-Tang to nourish blood and expel wind, disperse cold, and remove dampness	Green onion, garlic, coriander, parsley, fresh ginger, peppermint, Chinese chive, sunflower, celery
Kidney deficiency	Lower back pain, weak legs	Weakness of the legs, pain in the heel, light red tongue with a thin coating	Yang-Ying-Zhuang-Shen-Tang to strengthen the kidney	Abalone, chestnut, chicken, mutton, pork kidney, shrimp, string bean

FOOD CURE RECIPE

Cut up 2 pork kidneys and put black peppercorns inside them according to your age (1 corn for each year of age). Roast the kidneys and eat. This is particularly good for lower back pain associated with kidney deficiency.

SYNDROME	DISTINCT SIGNS	GENERAL SIGNS	HERBAL FORMULA	FOOD CURES
Blood coagulation	Pain all over the body or in the joints with stiffness or in the lower abdomen that intensifies on pressure	Intermittent abdominal pain, swelling, falling sensation in the lower abdomen, dark complexion, purple tongue	Shen-Tong-Zhu-Yu-Tang to nourish and activate blood, promote blood circulation, and relieve pain	Brown sugar, black soybean, chestnut, eggplant, ginger (fresh), papaya, sunflower, wine

LACK OF LACTATION AFTER CHILDBIRTH

Under normal circumstances, a woman's milk supply will be well established within three to four days after delivery. In some cases, the new mother suffers from lack of milk after delivery. This symptom may arise from the following two syndromes; each of them should be treated differently.

BLOOD DEFICIENCY: Blood is the source of milk. If a woman displays blood deficiency after delivery, she is bound to experience problems with milk supply.

LIVER ENERGY CONGESTION: A woman may experience emotional disturbances after delivery, particularly depression and anger, which affect the liver, causing liver energy congestion. This may lead to engorgement (uncomfortably full, hard breasts).

SYNDROME	DISTINCT SIGNS	GENERAL SIGNS	HERBAL FORMULA	FOOD CURE
Blood deficiency	No milk secretion or little secretion, clear, diluted milk	No swelling or pain in the breasts, pale complexion, poor appetite, fatigue	Tong-Ru-Dan to tone energy, nourish blood, and promote lactation	Azuki bean, beef, carp, chicken, day lily, lettuce, longan, octopus, peanuts, red date, tofu

FOOD CURE RECIPES

DAY LILY: Cut 60 g of pork into small pieces and steam it over water with 30 g of day lily. Eat at mealtime for one week as a course of treatment.

OCTOPUS: Cut up 120 g of fish and 2 pork feet and boil them in 2 cups (500 mL) of water until cooked. Season it with salt for consumption at mealtime. Repeat 3 to 5 times over the course of a week.

TOFU: Boil 20 g of tofu and 30 g of brown sugar in a cup of water over low heat for 10 minutes. Add 1 cup (250 mL) of wine for one-day consumption. Repeat 3 to 5 times.

PEANUTS: Cut up 2 pork feet and boil in 2 cups (500 mL) of water with 200 g of peanuts until cooked. Season it with salt, and divide into two portions for consumption at mealtimes. Repeat 3 times as a course of treatment.

SYNDROME	DISTINCT SIGNS	GENERAL SIGNS	HERBAL FORMULA	FOOD CURES
Liver energy congestion	Total absence of milk or only a little bit, swelling and pain in the breasts or hardness, concentrated and sticky milk	Poor appetite, low fever, emotional depression, decreased appetite, the tongue is dark red	Xia-Ru-Yong-Quan-San to disperse liver energy and promote lactation	Azuki bean, beef, bird's nest, button mushroom, rock sugar, sweet potato, sweet rice. Avoid pungent and spicy foods

FOOD CURE RECIPES

ORANGE PEEL: Cut up a pork foot and boil it in 2 cups (500 mL) of water with 20 g of orange leaves until cooked. Season with oil and salt, and eat at mealtime. Repeat 3 to 5 times as a course of treatment.

PAPAYA: Boil 500 g of papaya, 2 cups (500 mL) of rice vinegar, and 30 g of fresh ginger for 30 minutes. Divide into two doses for consumption at mealtime. Repeat twice.

INCONTINENCE OF MILK

Sometimes a mother will experience milk leaking from her breasts without sucking from the baby. This is called incontinence of milk and the symptoms do not include the following two normal occurrences: one, a new mother may be in good health with abundant energy and blood, so her breasts are full of milk that overflows; two, a mother's milk may overflow due to a delay in feeding the baby. This symptom may arise from the following two syndromes; each of them should be treated differently.

DEFICIENT ENERGY AND BLOOD: The body can function normally only with a sufficient quantity of energy and blood in it. When there is energy and blood deficiency, the body cannot control its own functions properly, so that the milk flows out right after its production. This means that the body is unable to store it for long.

HEAT CONGESTION IN THE LIVER MERIDIAN: The liver performs the excreting function. Emotional disturbances, stress, and anger in particular may cause liver energy congestion to generate heat in the liver. The heated liver performs its excreting function excessively, which causes the milk to overflow.

SYNDROME	DISTINCT SIGNS	GENERAL SIGNS	HERBAL FORMULA	FOOD CURE
Deficient energy and blood	Continual and natural flow of clear and diluted milk in small quantity, soft breasts with no swelling	Pale complexion, nervousness, palpitation, pale tongue with scanty coating on the tongue	Ba-Zhen-Tang to tone energy and blood simultaneously	Azuki bean soup, chicken soup, longan soup, red date

FOOD CURE RECIPES

GINSENG: Steam 10 g of ginseng to release the juice from it. Boil 60 g of rice in water until cooked. Pour the ginseng broth into the rice and mix them. Repeat 3 to 5 times over the course of a week.

MALT: Fry 120 g of malt for a minute or so, then add 2 cups of water and boil until cooked. Season with brown sugar for consumption anytime for 5 days as a course of treatment.

SYNDROME	DISTINCT SIGNS	GENERAL SIGNS	HERBAL FORMULA	FOOD CURE
Heat congestion in the liver meridian	Continual and natural flow of concentrated milk in large quantity, swollen and painful breasts	Congested chest, dry throat, bitter taste in the mouth, insomnia, dry stools, yellowish urine, red tongue with a thin layer of yellowish coating on the tongue	Dan-Zhi-Xiao-Yao-San to disperse the liver and clear heat	Abalone, celery, clam, crab, day lily, royal jelly, crab, jellyfish. Avoid pungent and spicy foods, sweet and greasy foods, which will increase phlegm

FOOD CURE RECIPES

WATER CHESTNUT: Peel 60 g of water chestnut, rinse 30 g of jellyfish in water. Boil the two ingredients in 2 cups (500 mL) of water until cooked. Season it with white sugar for consumption at mealtime, once a day for a week as a course of treatment.

FERMENTED BLACK SOYBEANS: Soak 100 g of rice in water for half an hour. Pour 1 tablespoon peanut oil into a frying pan to heat it up, add 3 tablespoons of fermented black soybeans, the rice, and 2 cups (500 mL) of water. Boil until cooked. Consume at mealtime, once a day for a week as a course of treatment.

CHAPTER 10

Treatment of Specific Disorders in Women

Women are yin and blood is their essence. —LI SHI ZHEN

This chapter covers premenstrual syndrome (PMS), infertility in women, perimenopause, menopause, and osteoporosis.

Premenstrual syndrome

Before your menstrual cycle starts each month, you may experience breast tenderness and cramps; you might feel anxious and irritable, depressed, exhausted, and bloated. Your mood may shift for no apparent reason, swinging between excitement and depression. You may experience weight gain, headache, or backache. These symptoms are referred to as premenstrual syndrome. The following are the three most common conditions behind most cases of PMS:

LIVER ENERGY CONGESTION: Toward the end of the menstrual cycle, you have more blood than normal, a condition that may cause liver energy congestion, creating excessive emotions. You may experience swelling and pain in your breasts to such a degree that your breasts cannot even touch your clothes without causing pain. You may also feel swelling and pain in your lower abdomen.

PHLEGM FIRE DISTURBING UPWARD: If your body contains more phlegm than usual, the phlegm may heat up gradually and turn into fire, causing excessive emotions.

DEFICIENT HEART BLOOD: When you have sufficient heart blood, your spirit will be well balanced. But when you have deficient heart blood, you may develop an emotional imbalance.

SYNDROME	DISTINCT SIGNS	SIGNS OF THE WHOLE BODY	HERBAL FORMULAS	FOOD CURES
Liver energy congestion	Feeling nervous, depressed, and anxious	Chest congestion, poor appetite, a thin, greasy coating on the tongue	Xiao-Yao-San or Chai-Hu-Shu-Gan-San or Dan-Zhi-Xiao-Yao-San	Beef, brown sugar, button mushroom, caraway seed, orange peel, spearmint, celery, yellow soybean, mung bean, eggplant, and cucumber
Phlegm fire disturbing upward	Feeling very irritable, headache, insomnia	Red face, pink eyes, congested chest, red tongue, yellow coating	Wen-Dan-Tang	Celery, seaweed, mung bean, corn, cucumber, seaweed, kelp
Deficient heart blood	Feeling depressed, incoherent speech, overdue menstruation	Poor spirits, insomnia, forgetfulness, nervousness, fatigue, easily in shock	Gan-Mai-Da-Zao-Tang with Yang-Xin-Tang	Chicken egg, wheat, rice, walnut, honey, ham, grape, potato, pork, and mutton

Treatment of infertility in women

Menstrual periods usually begin in a young girl's early teens or even earlier and continue until she is in her late forties or early fifties, when menstruation ceases (menopause). When menstruation occurs once a month without substantial change, it is called "monthly flood" in traditional Chinese medicine. In modern medicine, menstruation is regarded as the result of hormonal interactions, but in traditional Chinese medicine, it is regarded as resulting from interactions between kidney energy, innate kidney water, the vigorous meridian, and the conception meridian. A girl's kidney energy begins to activate at the age of seven and continues to build up until menopause. Kidney energy promotes the growth and development of the human body; it is stored between the two kidneys and as it develops, the innate kidney water in girls is activated to cause menstruation.

Both the rigorous and conception meridians originate in the womb; they play an essential role in menstruation and pregnancy. The conception meridian travels from the womb upward inside the abdomen to the throat. The vigorous meridian travels upward along the spinal column; it travels along the abdomen and meets the throat, then separates to link with the mouth and the lips. When the conception and vigorous meridians are disordered, female infertility can result. The menstrual cycles begin when the conception and vigorous meridians are full of energy and blood. After menstruation, these meridians possess more blood and energy, which is why women often display different physiological and psychological signs from their male counterparts.

Female infertility is treated mainly by Chinese herbs and acupuncture. When a couple consults a Chinese doctor of traditional medicine, the doctor will ask them questions, take their pulse, and examine their tongue to determine the causes of infertility. Once the cause is diagnosed, the TCM doctor will administer the appropriate herbal and acupuncture treatments. The Chinese have developed many dozens of herbal formulas and acupuncture points and techniques to treat infertility, and their success rates are remarkable. One reason for this success is that the Chinese people have put tremendous importance on fertility. If a person is infertile, it can be of great concern to this individual. Two thousand years ago Confucius said, "One can show filial disobedience in three ways, but failure to have children is the most serious one." Infertility is a great insult to a man, to say the least, and it can be a disaster for a woman.

Although acupuncture treatment of infertility has not been as successful as herbal treatment, it is a bona fide option. In fact, many celebrated Chinese classics of acupuncture have given considerable attention to this subject. The third-century *First Classic of Acupuncture and Moxibustion* says, "A woman with infertility and pain in the lower abdomen may be treated by the point located three fingers below the knee. A woman with infertility may be treated by the meeting point of triple yin energy. A childless woman should be treated by the bubbling fountain point." The *Compendium of Acupuncture and Moxibustion*, published in 1601, says, "A woman with infertility should be treated by the musical mountain point, the central extreme point. A woman without period, with yellowish complexion and infertility, should be treated by the bending pond point, the branching ditch point, the point three fingers below the knee, and the meeting point of the triple yin energy." All the points mentioned in these classic texts are common acupuncture points, familiar to all acupuncturists.

If you are a woman seeking treatment for infertility, the first thing is to make certain that your menstruation is normal; any existing menstrual disorder should be treated first. In one case, a childless 30-year-old female patient who had been married for over ten years and had never used contraceptives had given up hope of having a child. She went to a Chinese doctor and was treated for her menstrual disorders. To her surprise, a few months later, she was pregnant.

A well-known Chinese physician, Chen Xiu-Yuan (1753–1823), once said:

> *Female infertility may be attributed to menstrual disorders in most cases. Such disorders arise from a disturbance in the seven emotions, or the attack of the external pathogens, or imbalance in energy and blood, or a mutual attack between yin and yang forces. Thus, to treat female infertility means, in essence, to regulate the menstrual disorders. If, however, an infertile woman has normal menstrual cycles with no other illness, there are reasons to account for her infertility; one is obesity and the other is thinness.*

Among the many causes of female infertility, the following five are considered the most important contributing factors.

OBESITY

An obese woman, like an obese man, may appear strong on the outside but is really weak on the inside, and her weakness often contributes to her infertility. The most effective way of dealing with female infertility due to obesity is to reduce weight, which may be accomplished in three steps. First, reduce the quantity of water in the system, then tone up the energy conditions, and finally reduce the quantity of phlegm in the body. The treatment strategy is based on the theory that an obese woman suffers from three symptoms: too much water, too little energy, and too much phlegm in her body. Phlegm obstructs the free flow of energy and blood in the genital area, including the fallopian tubes. The treatment should be aimed at the above three symptoms and the formula Qi-Gong-Wan may be applied.

UNDERWEIGHT

A thin woman is full of fire and dryness in her system. Excessive fire will bring about deficient water, which is why her system is dry. A hot, dry body—like hot, dry soil—will not produce any offspring. The formula Yu-Lin-Zhu-Wan may be used to counteract dryness.

COLD WOMB

When a woman who is unable to become pregnant looks neither too fat nor too skinny, she is more likely to look pale or display symptoms of blood deficiency. Chances are that this type of woman cannot become pregnant due to a "cold womb," because there is not sufficient heat in her genitals required for fertilization—in the same way that we cannot plant seeds during the cold winter. A cold womb is more likely to prevent pregnancy by causing a blockage in the fallopian tubes.

It appears that very often there is a connection between frigidity and infertility in many women, but why does such a connection exist? Is it because a frigid woman has infrequent sexual intercourse, reducing her chances of pregnancy? On the surface, this seems to be the case, but in fact there is a deeper reason to explain the connection. A woman whose sexual organs are too cold may have frigidity and infertility at the same time. Just as a cold vagina cannot respond to sexual stimulus, so a cold womb cannot conceive a baby. The formula Wen-Bao-Yin may be used to treat both female infertility due to the cold womb and frigidity.

EMOTIONAL DISTURBANCES

If you cannot conceive for many years and you often experience premenstrual syndrome, irritability during menstruation, painful breasts before menstruation, and depression, chances are that you suffer liver energy congestion, and the formula Kai Yu Zhong Yu Tang may be used to restore your emotional balance. The English translation of this formula is "relieving the congestion and plant seeds decoction."

Some other commonly used formulas have been found effective for female infertility. Bu-Shen-Zhong-Zi-Wan ("toning the kidneys and planting the seeds tablets") is recommended for female infertility due to incomplete development of the uterus, irregular menstruation, and absence of ovulation. Bi-Fang-Zhong-Zi-Wan is recommended for female infertility due to cold womb, kidney deficiency, and blood coagulation. Tong-Luan-Shou-Yun-Zhong-Yu-Dan has shown success as well. Out of thirty-seven cases of female infertility due to fallopian blockage, twenty-five women became pregnant after this treatment.

In addition, acupuncture treatment of Guanyuan point (Ren 4), Zhongji point (R2), and the uterus point may be effective for inducing ovulation.

PAIN IN THE LOWER ABDOMEN

A woman may have been married for a long time but remains unable to conceive. Very often she may also display menstrual disorders with blood clots in menstrual flow and irregular menstruation. Shao-Fu-Zhu-Yu-Tang or Ge-Xia-Zhu-Yu-Tang may be used to treat this condition.

Two common causes of female infertility have been identified in Western medicine: failure to ovulate and blocked fallopian tubes. Traditional Chinese medicine has herbal formulas and acupuncture treatments to deal with both conditions.

Treatment of perimenopause

When a woman reaches her mid-forties through to mid-fifties, her monthly menstruation becomes irregular and then ceases. Her ovaries no longer function as before, and her estrogen secretion slows down and then stops. She may experience hot flashes, sudden chills, reduced vaginal lubrication, lowered sexual desire, emotional irritability, and sleeping disorders. This is called "perimenopause" or "menopause syndrome."

Menopause syndrome is closely related to the yin–yang imbalance in the kidneys and may last for two to three years. Menopause occurs as a result of the reduced production of kidney energy and innate kidney water, accompanied by a decline in the conception and vigorous meridians. However, bleeding that recurs after menstruation has stopped for a period of time is considered abnormal and requires careful diagnosis.

The symptoms of perimenopause may arise from the following two syndromes, which should be treated differently.

KIDNEY YIN DEFICIENCY: A woman may suffer chronic kidney yin deficiency syndrome either due to innate conditions or too many births or excessive sex. When she reaches her late forties, her kidney yin energy may decline further, which causes symptoms associated with kidney yin deficiency.

KIDNEY YANG DEFICIENCY: A woman suffers chronic kidney yang deficiency syndrome either due to innate conditions or too many births or excessive sex. When she reaches her late forties, her kidney yang energy may decline further, so that the kidneys cannot warm and transform water, which flows downward to cause flooding. That accounts for various symptoms arising from kidney yang deficiency.

SYNDROME	DISTINCT SIGNS	SIGNS OF THE WHOLE BODY	HERBAL FORMULA	FOOD CURES
Kidney yin deficiency	Hot flashes, vaginal dryness, mental depression, jumpiness, red face, perspiration, hot sensations in the center of the palms and the soles of the foot	Poor memory, poor concentration, anxiety, dizziness, ringing in the ears, insomnia, many dreams, backache, dry mouth, hard stools, decreased urination in yellowish color, red tongue with scanty coating on the tongue	Zuo-Gui-Wan to water the yin and soften the liver, rejuvenate yin energy and oppress yang energy to strike a balance	Wheat, red date, licorice, sweet rice, yam, honey, day lily. In case of hypertension, eat seaweed, celery, clam, and mussels to water yin and bring down fire
Kidney yang deficiency	Night sweats, dark complexion, poor spirits, chill, cold limbs	Poor appetite, abdominal swelling, watery stools, puffy face and limbs, frequent urination, incontinence of urination in severe cases, pale tongue with a thin layer of whitish coating	You-Gui-Wan to warm the kidneys and boost yang energy	In case of edema, reduce the intake of salt, eat more wintermelon, azuki bean, and cuttlefish soup. Avoid cold fruits, and other cold foods, such as mussels before and during menstruation

Treatment of osteoporosis

Osteoporosis results from the loss in bone density; bones become brittle and easily fracture, mostly as a result of aging. Women are more vulnerable to osteoporosis than men, particularly after menopause when the ovaries no longer produce estrogen hormones, which help maintain bone mass. Other causes are calcium deficiency and removal of the ovaries. In traditional Chinese medicine, it is believed that osteoporosis is due primarily to the deficiency of the spleen and the kidneys and reduction in blood and pure essence of the kidneys.

SYMPTOMS AND SIGNS	SYNDROMES AND TREATMENT
Pale tongue with white coating on the tongue, pain in the local region, fatigue, weak limbs, excessive perspiration, stomach discomfort	Blood deficiency and blood coagulation: Sheng-Ling-Bai-Zhu-San with Dang-Gui-Si-Ni-Tang, or Dang-Gui-Si-Ni-Tang with Da-Huang-Fu-Zi-Tang to strengthen the spleen and benefit energy
Red tongue with thin white coating on the tongue, blurred vision, cold hands and feet. Dizziness, dry sensations in the mouth particularly at night, dry throat, fatigue, hot sensations, night sweats, pain in the heel or tibia, retention of urine, ringing in ears, sleeplessness, thirst, toothache or loose teeth	Kidney yin deficiency: Zhi-Bai-Di-Huang-Wan to water the kidneys yin and strengthen bone

Index